STRONG
AFTER 60

The Seniors Strength Training Guide for Improved Energy, Mobility and Balance.

With a Home Exercise Plan!

By

Sophie Smith

I0134809

sophie@strongandstretchy.co.uk

DISCLAIMER

The information in this book is not intended to diagnose or treat any medical conditions. Always seek the advice of a medical professional before making drastic lifestyle changes. The author of this book accepts no liability for injury.

BEFORE YOU START!

Before you embark on your strength training journey I'd like to invite you to receive a **FREE 28 day Posture Improvement Plan!**

Just email 'Posture Plan' to sophie@strongandstretchy.co.uk and I'll send you your copy!

SOPHIE SMITH

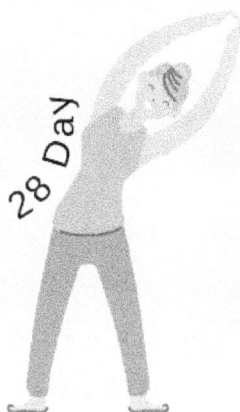

28 Day

POSTURE
PLAN

I'd also love to invite you to join our incredible Facebook community of over 60's taking control of their strength and independence, you can find us on Facebook at

'Strength Training and Stretches for Over 60s'

We will welcome you with open arms!

QR CODE
EXPLANATION

Throughout this book you'll find many QR codes, a code for each movement in fact! When you scan a QR code using the camera on your mobile phone, you will be able to watch a video of the movement being performed.

I've always found that a visual demonstration is the easiest way to understand a movement so I hope you find this feature useful.

If you don't have a camera phone don't worry, there's step by step instructions and illustrations to help you learn each movement!

Here's a QR code to help you practice viewing the videos:

Step 1. Open up the camera app on your phone.

Step 2. Hold your phone up to this QR code to scan it so that you can see the code on your screen. You'll see a small pop up saying 'Youtube' on your screen, click on that to watch the video!

TABLE OF CONTENTS

INTRODUCTION

By the time 65 rolls around, the last thing you want to be doing is worrying about healthcare, but that's exactly what you will be doing if you don't look after yourself, according to the stats. The average cost for healthcare is $11.3K a year in the United States for 65 year olds[i]. Yikes. Can you imagine working hard your whole life, only to have to fork out thousands for medical costs rather than living the lavish retirement that you've spent your whole life looking forward to? Retirement should be a little more exciting than days spent worrying and experiencing financial dismay. Other than getting a state-of-the-art private medical plan (and by "state-of-the-art", I mean the kind that requires you to trade an organ on the black market!), what else can you do?

Well, that's why I'm here, to tell you that there is a solution. And it's free and accessible to all. As an older adult, regular strength training is one of the most significant things you can do for your health. It can help you to become more mobile and strong for starters, then there's the simple yet oh-so-incredible fact that physical activity can deliver a powerful "get-out-and-stay-out" message to heart disease and diabetes, whilst giving your immune system a confidence boost! All of this means you're at less risk of becoming a burden to others or incurring expensive medical bills because of falls and other health complications, which translates to improved wellbeing and a longer, happier life.

I imagine that you chose this book because you feel and see the signs of aging, and you may be experiencing a sense of helplessness. Maybe the telltale aches, pains, and physical manifestations of what is often associated as part of getting older are becoming a little harder to "just ignore".

You woke up this morning, and suddenly, the stairs on the second floor seemed a little steeper, joint pain has become an inconvenient norm, and range of motion might seem like it's gone on an unauthorized vacation.

But the good news is, this isn't your forever reality. In fact, all of these issues likely aren't even effects of aging, but rather effects of prolonged inactivity. And we're about to get active alright!

I am here to help you become the strongest, healthiest version of yourself so that you can maintain a quality of life that has you eager to get out of bed in the morning. There's so much living left to do, and with a strong and healthy body, you can do just that!

As a strength training enthusiast, I know that small changes can have a big impact, and according to a study published in Science Daily[ii], seniors who partake in strength training just twice a week have a significant increase in quality of life and a lower mortality risk - now that sounds like a good incentive to me!

According to motivational speaker and author Mel Robbins, the odds of us being born are one in 400 trillion. I don't believe that decades of this rare, precious gift of life should be wasted due to fear of falling, having physical pain, or no energy. We weren't given this gift to not enjoy it!

But why allow me to help you? Well, I'm a qualified sports massage therapist with qualifications in senior fitness. I have years of experience studying human anatomy and have worked with a range of muscle imbalances, motivational blocks and fitness levels both with my clients and on my own body.

But it's not just little old me here to help you, I've also recruited my good friend Chris Thompson who just so happens to be a military Exercise Rehabilitation Instructor with over 15 years' experience of fixing bodies just like yours. He has created a strength training plan just for you, because you deserve the very best!

It would be one thing to tell you that my driving inspiration and passion for this book stemmed from my love of fitness and helping others. That is true, but it's about much more than that for me. It also stems from my aging parents.

I've always had a burning desire to give my parents the best life possible, and for the most part the overwhelming thought in my mind has been, "Once I make a certain amount of money, I can take my parents on nice holidays and treat them to nice things." While this is still on my goals list, it hit me a few years ago that the biggest gift I can give them is to help them maintain their health and fitness. *That* will be what truly inspires a quality life for them.

If you can't walk on a beach or climb up castle steps or get up off a sunbed, going on holiday won't bring much joy at all! The same applies to daily life; it pains me to see older adults struggling to play with their grandchildren, or losing their independence and strength as they age as if it's a given as the years go on. I'm here to tell you it's not a given, and there are seniors out there living full, long, strong independent lives.

Since having this realization, I knew that senior health and fitness would be what I would throw myself into for the years to come. I can place my hand on my heart and say that nothing makes me more content than seeing someone who thought they'd never feel strong again, feel powerful, confident and shocked at just how much they can still achieve.

If I can help even just one person reading this book to have that "I can't wait to get out of bed and live today" feeling, because they're no longer in pain and feel physically strong and energetic, all of my years of studying and writing will be worth it.

My goal is that this book motivates you to make the most of this wonderful life, showing you that it's not difficult or unrealistic to feel strong and energetic once again. I want this book to be a symbol of hope that your life is not over. This is a new, exciting chapter that you're yet to enjoy and it's never too late to start a new journey.

So, without any more rambling on from me, let's get started!

TOPICS DISCUSSED

Though my hope is that the first time you pick up this book, you read through it all, I understand that some of you will be here simply to gain certain pieces of information. Maybe you've forgotten how much you should be eating to get stronger, in which case you could flick to the 'Fuel' chapter. Or maybe you just need some inspiration for some great movements to try out, in which case you could flick to the movement glossary. To help you navigate through this book in the most efficient way, I've included a list below of what is explored throughout with the page number to match so you can quickly find what you need.

Laying the Foundations (PART 1, PAGE 12)

Some might say that what you do to your body, you do to your mind. So it would make sense that 'losing your marbles' for want of a better phrase, is directly linked to your exercise habits or lack thereof! That's why it's important to have a holistic approach to taking care of your physical, mental, and emotional states. Think of exercise as one of those "all-inclusive" deals - when you exercise, it creates balance in all of these areas. This section of the book covers the benefits of strength training, mind, body and soul.

Fuel (PART 1, PAGE 26)

We've all heard the saying, 'you are what you eat', and at the risk of sounding like an annoying broken record, it's true. If you eat rubbish, your workout results will be rubbish, and your mood and general wellbeing probably will be too. Sorry, but as brutal as that sounds, it's the truth (packs muffins away surreptitiously!) Just like you wouldn't fuel your car with sludge, you shouldn't fuel your body with incorrect foods before or after a workout or any day in between. It's essential to get enough water, vitamins, nutrients, and plenty of sleep to be the best, healthiest version of you! As a lover of pizza and donuts and really any carbs myself, I'm not for one second telling you it's salad from here on out (are we friends again now?). But moderation is key. Providing you're fueling your body with enough of the nutrient rich food you need, treats are always encouraged in moderation because this is about changing your lifestyle, not restricting you so much that it's easy to fall back into old unhealthy ways. This section of the book will provide you with some basic nutritional guidelines to keep you running!

Mobility and Warming Up (PART 2, PAGE 35)

Our busy lifestyles mean we often look for shortcuts and I've been guilty of doing this in my workouts before by skipping my warmup. But this little 'shortcut' sets you on a dangerous path that can lead to injuries and even more pains and niggles (trust me, I've done the trial and error for you!).

Warming up is essential to get the most out of your strengthening exercises and to avoid injury. In this section of the book I will ensure that you're equipped with everything you need to know about getting your body warmed up, supple, and raring to go for an effective workout!

Strength Training Program (PART 2, PAGE 48)

Every 5-star meal requires the right ingredients and a tried-and-tested recipe. It's much the same with your workouts. You may understand the movements but won't get the full benefit from them if you don't know how to put them together to create an effective strength training session. To help you understand how to do this, or to save you the work if you don't want to figure out how, I have worked with my previously mentioned good friend and military Exercise Rehabilitation Instructor to create workouts perfectly suited to the 60+ age group. But before you worry that you're about to be expected to march, hop, skip and jump to the tune of a drill sergeant, you'll be pleased to know that while each workout is created with building strength in mind, they also focus on mobility and improving your balance and energy levels. Your strength training lifestyle isn't supposed to feel like a punishment, it's a celebration of all your incredible body can (still) do. In this section of the book your strength training lifestyle will begin.

Cool down and Stretches (PART 2, PAGE 83)

Just as there is a time for moving and shaking your body maraca-style into shape, there's also a time to chill out, stretch, and cool down. This is so that the exercise you've just exposed your muscles to has the time to do its good work, because rest and relaxation is needed for growth (and sanity). In this section you'll be provided with a cool down sequence and some stretches to help you feel flexible and ready for the rest of your day.

Glossary of Strength Training Exercises (PART 2, PAGE 101)

Once you've used the provided exercise plans to build your strength and improve your mobility and balance, you don't need to stop there. I've also included a nifty exercise glossary, which is a valuable tool to refer to when you're ready to create your own exercise routines. In this glossary, you will find some key compound movements and a number of uncomplicated accessory movements to bring a bit of variety and pizazz into your workouts. Because who needs a boring workout, right?

Tailored Workouts (PART 2, PAGE 160)

In this chapter you'll find a variety of workouts to try! Some have been specifically created to help with a certain area of weakness, like a weak back for example. Others have been created to help with a certain ailment, like Sciatica pain. And 30 have been created to help improve your strength, balance and mobility! With this wealth of workout inspiration your strength training journey never needs to get boring!

PART 1

LAYING THE FOUNDATIONS

It is never too late to make a change. Whether you have been sedentary all your life or have just fallen off the wagon, there is still time to make an incredible transformation, both physically and mentally, even if, at the moment, it feels as though the wagon rode over you a few times!

Exercise is one of the most important things we can do for our health. It can prevent and slow down many of the health problems that may come with age and prolong our quality of life.

In Part 1 we will be exploring the holistic benefits of strength training and learning how to build strong foundations for a long, happy fitness journey.

Part 1. Chapter 1.

EXERCISE AND THE BRAIN

"Exercise not only tones the muscles, but also refines the brain and revives the soul" - Michael Treanor

Most of us know that exercise is beneficial for the mind because of the "feel-good" chemicals that are released during a workout. When we are physically active, our bodies release endorphins, which are the body's natural pain killer and mood elevator. These endorphins interact with the receptors in our brain to reduce our perception of pain. They also trigger a positive sensation in the body, similar to the feeling of morphine. While they won't leave you floating on a morphine-infused fluffy-pink cloud, they are scientifically proven mood boosters, enhancing feelings of happiness and euphoria.

Even moderate exercise a few times a week produces these happy-buzz-infusing endorphins, which, when combined with other factors, can significantly improve anxiety and depression. Such is the improvement that doctors may recommend trying out an exercise regime before turning to medication (the good doctors, anyway).

You've likely already heard of endorphins, and I'm sure you know that exercise is good for you, or you wouldn't be here reading this book! But did you know that exercise affects more than just endorphin release and physical strength? According to psychologist and biostatistician Patrick J. Smith[iv], physical activity triggers the release of a protein called brain-derived neurotrophic factor. BDNF is an important molecule in the brain that encourages the growth of new cells through neurogenesis. This could include the hippocampus, a region in the brain vital for memory and learning. Neurogenesis improves overall brain performance and prevents memory loss and cognitive decline by strengthening the hippocampus. One fear of some older adults is quite literally losing their minds, either through dementia or Alzheimer's. So I hope you can find comfort in the fact that your new strength training routine is scientifically proven to be beneficial for your brain and could prevent these horrible conditions.

Researchers have even proven that six months of lifting weights can help protect the brain, especially the areas vulnerable to Alzheimer's, for up to one year later. And another study published in the Archives of Internal Medicine[v] states that exercise programs involving weight training could help stave off progression to dementia in seniors who are already showing signs of cognitive impairment. I hope this motivates you even more to get started with building your body and your brain!

Exercise boosts our brainpower in so many ways; it's a wonder it's not prescribed by every doctor. Mores the pity, it doesn't come in tablet form! What a great way to ensure you get enough exercise; simply pop the exercise pill of choice, running, yoga, etc. Then lie down for a nice nap, and hey presto! Exercise done, abs formed, muscles worked! But back to the point I was trying to make. Studies have also shown that physical exercise boosts our creativity and mental energy levels. So, if you are in need of inspiration, your big idea could be just a workout away!

And then there's those pesky stress levels. Exercise also reduces these, which in this often-chaotic world, is something we could all use! By safely increasing our heart rate, we can even reverse stress-induced brain damage by stimulating the production of neurohormones like norepinephrine. These hormones improve our mood and cognition and enhance our thinking when clouded by stressful scenarios. I know this all sounds too good to be true, but I promise you I'm not making these long fancy words up, this is science talking!

Next on the list of things that often deteriorate with age are self-esteem and self-confidence. In fact, one of the most upsetting things I see in my massage clients, and as the daughter of a 'senior' (sorry, Mom), is the complete lack of self-love and confidence in many older people. Suddenly age makes many see their bodies through un-tinted glasses, and the picture is far from rosey!

It's almost as though there is a lack of appreciation for the body. This vessel that has carried you through decades, through recessions, heartbreak, hormone changes, new jobs, not to mention the strains of having kids (physical and mental), is suddenly unvalued. The only thing many older adults seem to see is a body that isn't as tight or strong as it used to be. Enter the deflated balloon identity crisis, as I like to call it.

But when you use strength training to realize your potential and see evidence that you're still capable of more than you could possibly imagine, it can lead to a massive boost in self-esteem and confidence. Of course, your goal may not be to become a bikini model (although I'll be here cheering you on if it is!) or to set a weightlifting world record (although that is still totally possible, honestly!). But improving your ability to get up the stairs without losing your breath, Darth Vader style, play with your grandchildren on the floor, or wake up feeling refreshed and filled with purpose are all mighty wins in themselves. These simple actions combined can make you love and appreciate yourself and your life in the way you should.

So I guess what I'm trying to say is that there really is no downside to exercising, but there's an unlimited number of potential benefits - for your body, brain and soul!

Part 1. Chapter 2.

EXERCISE AND THE BODY

"Exercise is a celebration of what your body can do. Not a punishment." - Anon

Exercising is not just about looking good or feeling great, although both those things are an added bonus. More importantly, it's about looking after the future you. Our lean muscle naturally diminishes with age, and strength training is the best solution to prevent this from happening.

Strength training can help us preserve and enhance our muscle mass at any age. Sarcopenia (muscle atrophy) may sound like the latest Alien vs Predator movie title but it is actually a natural aging process where the body experiences age-related muscle loss. After the age of thirty, we begin to lose as much as 3% to 5% of muscle per decade. It's scary to think this natural process automatically kicks in and quietly saps at our muscle strength. Obviously, this results in less muscle on the body, which means we have less mobility and more significant weakness, leaving our bones and joints less supported. This, in turn, increases our risk of fractures and falls. In addition, weak muscles can affect anything from walking or climbing stairs to having back or neck ache. But, I'm sure you know this and probably feel it, which is likely why you're here!

However, something that isn't common knowledge is how specific muscle weakness can negatively impact the whole body. My clients often look at me as though I'm psychic when I run tests with them and suggest that their back pain could be due to a seemingly unrelated muscle. This is because our bodies need balance to operate efficiently and remain pain-free; if that balance is out of whack, it impacts other parts of the body. This is why I can almost certainly say that if you have a niggle right now, it could be due to a muscle imbalance you've never even considered; no crystal ball required!

Let's take a look at what could be causing your back pain as an example.

1. **Weak glutes**

   Strong glutes are essential for the health of our lower back since they assist with our pelvic, hip, and trunk motions. Now you know where the term 'buns of steel' comes from! The glutes also help to evenly distribute the load throughout our lower back and lower extremities and assist with good posture. So if you're experiencing back pain, it could in fact be down to your glute muscles not firing properly!

2. **A weak core**

   Back pain is common in people with a weak core. When your abdominal muscles are weak, your back muscles have to over compensate. So building good core strength will help bring balance and harmony to the front and back of your body. A stronger core can also lead to less chance of compressed discs in your spine due to sitting all day. I bet you never guessed that sitting and doing nothing physical all day could be a dangerous alternative to exercise!

3. **Tight hip flexors**

   When sitting for long periods of time, your back could become sore due to your psoas muscle (a hip flexor) being shortened and pulling on your lower back.

The Good News..

This example shows that the pain or difficulty experienced when completing certain tasks that you blame on just "getting older" could actually be the product of a weak muscle lurking somewhere you haven't even considered. It also shows why treating the area you feel the pain in may also not solve the issue, but strengthening your muscles so that they can work in harmony, can.

The body is so intricately connected that by strengthening certain muscles, you can feel like a new, stronger version of you who can enjoy life and all it has to offer again. Besides, who needs the fountain of youth when you have exercise on your side?

And as I've just mentioned youth, I'd like to tackle another common belief; that it's too late to make a real difference to these pains and niggles now that you're a 'senior'. This couldn't be further from the truth. When talking about exercise, Exercise Physiologist Jeff Payne doesn't believe that any specific age exists. He explains, "I've trained some 70-year-olds that move like 40-year-olds, and I've definitely trained some 40-year-olds that move like 70-year-olds". So while you will lose some muscle mass due to aging, there's still plenty of time to turn things around and prevent your muscle aches and pains by strengthening your body!

Why else is it important for over 60s to get physically stronger?

Reducing aches and pains isn't the only benefit of strength training as we age, many of the common concerns and ailments experienced amongst older adults could also be prevented through following a good training program. As a 'senior', you don't need to be a competitive weightlifter (unless you want to be), but the more powerful your muscles are, the healthier and happier you will be. Here's why:

1. **Stronger muscles reduce the risk of falls.**

   Sadly, fall-related injuries are very common among seniors and are often very serious. You wouldn't believe the injuries that occur amongst older adults completing simple tasks like watering the garden, vacuuming, or even carrying a cup of tea. Suddenly, these simple tasks require the same level of dexterity as seen in a Jacki Chan film, and it's often simply down to instability resulting from weakened muscles. Performing exercises to strengthen your muscles just two or three times a week can significantly improve your muscle imbalances, meaning there's less risk of falls or injuries. Studies have shown that even a basic strength training routine can increase bone density, balance, and overall strength which means you can continue living your daily life without the fear of falling or injuring yourself.

2. **Strength training fights osteoporosis.**

As we age, our bone density decreases. This can lead to osteoporosis, where the bones are more prone to breaks and fractures because they become brittle and soft. Several studies have shown that strength training can slow bone loss and even build bone. This means that your new strength training lifestyle should actually improve your bone strength and density which can help to offset age related bone mass decline.

3. **Stronger muscles fight osteoarthritis.**

Osteoarthritis is a condition where the cartilage between the joints breaks down as we age. It causes pain, stiffness, and loss of movement in the joints. Strength training can effectively combat osteoarthritis and improve joint mobility, and it's not just me saying this, results from 8 different studies of older adults with osteoarthritis reported a pain reduction of 35% when partaking in a strength training program. Movement is magic!

It's Never Too Late to Transform your Body

After learning just how much the body is connected and the hugely positive impact strength training can have, you may be beating yourself up for the fact that you're only just starting, or are only just getting back into it if you've neglected training for a few years. But please don't worry, it is truly never too late to start.

A study published by Frontier in Physiology[vi] discovered some motivating results that will hopefully reassure you of the progress you can still make. There were two groups of people involved. One group consisted of seventy to eighty year olds who had been exercising their entire lives. The other group consisted of people who had never trained seriously (semi-couch potatoes!). Scientists gave each group the same workout and gave each person an isotope tracer to drink before the session. Muscle biopsies were taken before and after the workout to discover how their muscles responded and to everyone's surprise, the proteins in the muscles of the untrained and trained individuals both demonstrated the same potential to grow.

It may be intimidating to think about starting a new strength training routine as an older adult, but this study demonstrates that even if you haven't led a gym-worshipping lifestyle, you can still make serious progress by starting now! In fact, this shows you that it's entirely possible to transform your body for the better without having ANY prior training experience. So there is no excuse not to start right now!

Part 1. Chapter 3.

EXERCISE AND THE SOUL

"I hate how you get older, and society seems to see you as weak and incapable. I still enjoy LOUD Rock n' Roll music, being active and having fun. I'm the same person, just in an older body. Thankfully, I'm lucky enough to believe that. But I can see a lot of people don't because society paints older people as non-productive, not fully functioning people who are no longer worthy enough to live a fun life. Just look at those awful road signs; older people are painted as hunched over with a walking stick! It's no wonder many people accept that as they get older, they'll automatically become more fragile and less competent, and that's a really sad belief."
- The words of one of my favorite 'seniors'.

Many things in life are beyond our control and getting older is one of them. But by choosing to exercise, you are making the decision to take back control of your life. Strength training can help prevent you from becoming 'one of those' stereotypical seniors with a walking stick and no purpose! The truth is, fragility doesn't need to be your reality just because your age is increasing. And another thing that shouldn't fade with age, is your enjoyment of life.

The way I like to look at strength training is as a celebration of the body and all it can do. It's also a way for me to become engulfed in my favorite music and forget about the stresses in my daily life and I hope it becomes the same for you. Done right, an exercise routine is a party without the hangover!

Exercise is also a great way to get out of the house and get social. Older age can be lonely for many people, so working out in a group or even at the park can reduce those feelings of loneliness and bring some happiness to your soul. And if, like me, you prefer to workout alone, the strength you'll gain from your sessions will help you stay active and mobile for the years to come. This means you get to continue doing the things you love with the people you love for a long time!

Exercise shouldn't be a chore; we have enough of those! Instead, my goal is to help you enjoy your workouts, and for them to be the highlight of your day or week as you honor everything you are capable of.

I want your training sessions to involve feeling good on every level, physically, mentally, and spiritually. So, turn up your favorite music, dance like it's your birthday every day and make your workout a party more than a chore! Because the ability to move truly is worth celebrating.

Summary

Phew! You made it! Though these chapters were information heavy, I feel having the knowledge behind *why* you should strength train is important. If you ever feel like giving up, you can now remind yourself of all of the reasons to continue.

   The key takeaways from these chapters are:
   - Staying strong and healthy is often overlooked, but it is essential to ensuring a good quality of life. Strength training benefits us holistically and in every way, I really am yet to hear of a downside.
   - Strong muscles support our body's ability to effectively accomplish what we need to in our everyday lives and reduce our risk of injury and pain.

- Getting older doesn't mean you are no longer able to exercise. You are completely capable of making a positive change, and it's so crucial for your general well-being.

In the next chapter, we will be talking about nutrition and looking after your body from the inside out. But don't worry, I won't be telling you it's all salad and water from here on out, we can still be friends!

Part 1. Chapter 4.

FUEL

"Exercise is king. Nutrition is queen. Put them together and you've got a kingdom" - Jack Lalanne.

Sufficient sleep and good nutrition are two important parts of getting strong and living your best possible life. However, before you yawn and slam the book shut, I promise they're not as boring or complicated as they may seem. In this chapter you'll be provided with all of the information you need to lay the best possible foundations for your strength training journey. And don't worry, I'm not one of those motivational fitness gurus who will tell you that even smelling sugar is a crime, we're all about balance over here. Oh, and I love to sleep, so I won't be depriving you of that, either!

Nutrition

Good nutrition is essential, no matter how old we are. Food fuels our bodies for the activities we need to complete daily. Without eating nutritionally balanced foods, our energy supplies are sporadic, leaving us feeling lethargic and unmotivated. Good nutrition may even prevent diseases like high blood pressure, diabetes, osteoporosis, and heart problems. And since getting older is linked to changes that make us prone to deficiencies in vitamin D, calcium, iron, vitamin B12, magnesium, and several other essential nutrients, maintaining a healthy diet throughout our lives is super important, especially as we get older.

Energy

I have tried and tested so many different restrictive diets, and they have always ended up in three things: misery, burnout, and binge eating. Life is meant for living, so enjoy it by eating your favorite foods in moderation, but not to the point where they're hindering your health or making you feel groggy. I get a tremendous sense of enjoyment from eating yummy food, and I will never stop indulging in that pleasure as long as it doesn't negatively impact my health, and neither should you! But remember that food is energy, and if it's not making you feel energized, you're probably eating the wrong types, or amounts! Let's look into this a little more..

Why nutrition is so important as we age, especially when adding in an exercise routine:

- Poor nutrition weakens your muscles and bones, leaving you vulnerable to injury, falling, and loss of independence. Protein aids the body in building, maintaining, and repairing healthy bones and muscles, so without sufficient amounts in your diet you could find yourself becoming weak and frail.
- Poor nutrition also leads to fatigue and lethargy, and even sometimes anemia. Good food is fuel for your body and without it your energy levels will be low, cue, one very grouchy you.
- And then there's the mood swings and emotional disorders often caused by poor nutrition. If you aren't getting enough nutrients into your body, it may have difficulty producing vital chemicals and hormones. For example, many foods like oily fish, beans, oats, and fresh berries trigger the production of dopamine and serotonin (the body's mood-enhancing chemicals), so including a variety of nutrient dense food in your diet can literally make you happier!

- Poor nutrition can also lead to digestive issues such as constipation or diarrhea. It is super important to consume enough fiber and whole grains and stay hydrated to prevent this.

So, what nutritional guidelines should you follow to ensure you stay healthy?

- Eat a wide variety of foods from the five food groups. These include plenty of colorful fruits, vegetables, legumes, beans, whole grains, high fiber cereals, lean meats and poultry, fish, tofu, eggs, seeds and nuts, yogurt, milk, and reduced-fat cheese or their alternatives. Try to get as many different colors on your plate when constructing your meals.
- Limit foods high in saturated fat like cakes, biscuits, pastries, pies, processed meats, fast food, crisps, and other savory snacks. Everything in moderation.
- Replace foods that are high in saturated, polyunsaturated, and monounsaturated fats. Swap cream, cooking margarine, and palm oil with fats from oils and spreads like olive oil, nut butter, healthy pastes, and avocado.
- Limit foods and drinks that contain added sugars like cordials, fruit juices, sports drinks, and sodas.
- Make sure to drink enough water and incorporate some physical activity into your day, even if you're not strength training. This could even be a couple of short walks just to get the blood flowing.

Estimated Daily Caloric Requirements for Older Adults

Females over 60
- Sedentary: 1,600 calories
- Moderately Active: 1,800 calories
- Active: 2,000-2,200 calories

Males over 60:
- Sedentary: 2,000-2,200 calories
- Moderately Active: 2,200-2,400 calories
- Active: 2,400-2,800 calories

Many online calculators can help to calculate your estimated daily calorie intake; however, it is important to keep in mind that factors like weight, height, obesity, etc., should be considered. Type this address into the search engine on your computer to get a free calculation: https://www.calculator.net/calorie-calculator.html.

It is advised to speak to your healthcare practitioner to get a more personalized calorie target because, after all, we are all unique and have different nutritional requirements. Once you start your strength training routine I would recommend aiming for the 'moderately active' calorie intake option for your gender, unless you have a physically demanding job in which case you'd choose the 'active' option.

One important factor regarding our calorie intake, is how much of that is from protein sources. Protein is the building blocks of our muscles and as soon as you're strength training regularly, you'll need to eat a sufficient amount of protein to build those muscles up! A good general guideline for protein intake is 0.8 - 1 grams of protein per pound of bodyweight. So if you weigh 145 lbs, you would want to consume between 116-145 grams of protein per day, with the majority of the rest of your diet consisting of high quality carbohydrates to give you sufficient energy (around 40-60%), and the rest of your food being healthy fats (around 20-30%). Pick a figure in between the 0.8-1 gram per body weight and trial it. Everyones body responds differently to protein so as long as you're hitting the minimum recommended amount, you can make small adjustments once you get used to how much your body needs.

Vitamins

As well as hitting your basic caloric goals and eating nutritious food daily, it is important that you are getting all the vitamins and minerals you need. Supplementation is often recommended and even necessary for older adults, so I suggest speaking to your doctor, who can help you calculate your specific needs.

Here is a list of seven supplements and vitamins that are great for the aging population!

1. Mushrooms

Mushrooms are a superfood! They are a delicious source of vitamin D and also contain B vitamins as well as potassium! The level of vitamin D varies with each type of mushroom like portobello, shiitake, chanterelle, and morel. Some mushroom supplements you can buy have been exposed to UV light to give them an even higher concentration of vitamin D. It's easy to add mushrooms to pasta dishes, omelets, and salads!

2. Garlic

Most people I know love garlic, and it's good for more than just flavoring food. Garlic is valuable for decreasing cholesterol and blood sugar, removing heavy metals from the body, acting as an antiviral and antifungal agent, and potentially preventing cancer. Garlic contains vitamins A, B, and C, iodine, potassium, selenium, iron, zinc, calcium, and magnesium.

3. Vitamin B6 and B12

These vitamins help the body make energy from the food we eat and form red blood cells, which carry oxygen throughout our bodies. B6 and B12 can be found in beef liver, mackerels, nutritional yeast, or shiitake mushrooms, but a vitamin B6 or B12 supplement is often needed because we don't get enough through our food. One of the symptoms of B12 deficiency is neurological problems, so some older folks have been able to improve their memory by getting an adequate amount of B12. It's definitely worth a try!

4. Honey

Honey is nature's nectar. It contains vitamins B6, C, calcium, and niacin and is packed with antioxidants. Some research shows that honey can also help combat anxiety and memory decline.

5. Vitamin K

A recent multi-ethnic study[viii] found that adults between the ages of 54 and 76 with low circulating vitamin K levels were more likely to pass away within 13 years than those with adequate levels. This study suggests that vitamin K may offer protective health benefits as we age. The most common foods with high levels of vitamin K are green leafy vegetables like spinach, kale, broccoli, cabbage, lettuce, and collard greens.

6. Calcium

As we age, there is a combination of inadequate intestinal absorption of calcium and age-related hormone decline, which adversely affects our bone health. Getting the proper calcium intake can reduce the risk of osteoporosis, fractures, and diabetes. The best sources of calcium are from supplements, poppy seeds, chia seeds, cheese, yogurt, sardines, beans and lentils, and almonds.

7. Vitamin C

Vitamin C has been proven to help neutralize free radicals in our bodies that lead to oxidative stress. This aids in preventing premature skin aging and delays the visible signs of biological aging. One of the best sources of vitamin C is Acerola Powder which is derived from the acerola cherry and has 65 times the vitamin C of an orange! Other vitamin C options are citrus, guavas, sweet yellow pepper, kiwis, brussel sprouts, and litchis.

Water

The sensation of thirst decreases with age, so it may be more challenging for older adults to tell when dehydration is on the horizon. Drinking enough water is vital because it keeps our electrolytes balanced, our blood volume normal, aids in digestion and the transportation of nutrients, and helps the kidneys to function properly. Becoming dehydrated can lead to mental confusion and other health consequences.

Here is a general daily fluid intake recommendation:
- **Approximately 15.5 cups (3.7 liters) a day for men**
- **Approximately 11.5 cups (2.7 liters) a day for women**

Around 20% of this water intake can come from the vegetables and fruit we eat daily. So aiming for the commonly recommended eight glasses of water a day should keep you sufficiently hydrated. Unfortunately, we are not like the humble camel capable of storing water in a handy hump (maybe this is fortunate on second thoughts!). So if you feel thirsty, you may have left it too long between drinks (of water, not gin!). A good way to ensure you remain hydrated is to drink water regularly throughout the day, by spreading your water intake, and you will easily reach the required eight glasses a day. When partaking in a strength training program it's recommended to drink even more to replenish after sweating, but the great thing about exercising is it makes you want to drink more anyway - another great reason to start!

Sleep

Sleep is a vital mechanism, regardless of our age. It has the ability to restore our energy levels and heal both cognitive and physical damage. Seven to eight hours of quality sleep per night is recommended to help us function at our best. The good news is that if you are someone who struggles to get a good night's sleep, your new exercise routine could help! A recent study[vii] has shown that in as little as four weeks, people who suffer from chronic insomnia, who began exercising regularly, could fall asleep up to 13 minutes faster and stay asleep 18 minutes longer. That's a whole half-hour of extra snooze time! Forget counting sheep; a good workout could give you the best and longest time in dreamland!

Summary

Fueling your body doesn't have to be an overly complicated process overseen by sciency-gurus. It's pretty simple, really, as it's just about balancing nutritious food and the right amount of sleep and hydration with your new exercise routine.

Please keep in mind that this chapter is merely to inform you about the importance of proper nutrition and is not intended to diagnose. It is always essential to seek the advice of your health care practitioner before drastically changing your diet or taking new supplements.

In the next chapter, you'll be getting that body moving!

PART 2

YOUR STRENGTH TRAINING GUIDE

"Aging is not lost youth but a new stage of opportunity and strength"
- Betty Friedan.

In Part 2 of this book you will find all the exercises you need to become a stronger you. You're about to embark on a strength training journey that has the potential to positively impact you in every way and I truly can't wait for you to surprise yourself with just how much your body is capable of, no matter how old or inactive you may currently be. You've got this!

Part 2. Chapter 5.

MOBILITY AND WARMING UP

The purpose of a warm-up is quite literally to *warm us up* before our workout. It is also the chance to prepare ourselves mentally and physically for the activity ahead. I often think that mentally readying ourselves for exercise is the hardest part of the warm-up routine! Our mischievous minds are adept at reminding us of our favorite tv program that's about to start or that cold glass of wine waiting to be poured in the kitchen. Unfortunately, most of us humans seem to prefer the path of least resistance and more relaxation! So it's totally normal to have to talk yourself into getting up to move, especially if this is a new journey for you.

But one great thing about getting up - that's the hardest bit done! Once you're up and moving with your favorite tunes on, I bet you'll soon be in the mood for more movement.

Warm-ups aren't just great for mentally getting us ready to exercise, but they're also like adding oil to a machine; they improve our mobility and increase our muscle elasticity so that we can exercise more efficiently. This prevents those dastardly muscle strains and pains!

Think of it like this:

If you're working on a computer and walk away to make some tea, the computer monitor might go to 'sleep.' Then, when you return to work, you have to move the mouse around to let the computer know you're back before you can start asking it to do a million things. It's the same with our bodies and warm-ups. Warming up is priming your body to be ready for a workout, so you get more value from the activity you are doing.

The benefits of warm-ups:

1. **A good warm-up slowly increases your heart rate, minimizing stress on your heart.** An increased heart rate also boosts blood flow, which increases body temperature. This enables more oxygen to reach your muscles, raising the temperature of the muscles for optimal efficiency. This results in your muscles contracting and relaxing easily, allowing you to perform more strenuous tasks with ease.

2. **Warming up also reduces the risk of injury.** The last thing you want when you're just getting into the swing of things is to become injured. Warming up will improve your muscle elasticity which means there's less chance of accidentally hurting yourself during your exercise session!

3. **Warming up engages the nervous system.** Your body and brain are constantly exchanging electrical signals. This is how you move, think and live. Of course, there are automatic functions that our bodies inevitably do, like breathing, but for intentional movement, you want to prime and engage your nervous system to be more responsive in order to produce the most efficient workout possible. By warming up you're increasing motor neuron recruitment and kickstarting your coordination!

Motivation tip: If you really don't feel like working out today, tell yourself you'll just do this warm-up so that you're doing something to move. Put on your favorite music with the purpose of just doing this one thing, and within a few minutes of moving, I bet you'll want to do more. This works for me everytime I'm having a 'I might just stay in bed today' day.

Basic Mobility/Warm-up

The following daily 5-10 minute warm-up sequence will prepare your joints and muscles for your workout. It can also help increase energy and blood flow all over the body. It can be used as a stand alone bout of exercise if you just need a quick refresher during the day or as a warm-up before an exercise session. This warm-up is universal and can be used before all of the workouts in this book.

Once you are more advanced in your strength training journey, potentiation is great to add onto your warmups after this sequence. Potentiation is about getting your body ready to perform, and your neuromuscular system switched on to move fast. It's performing movements that you'll be including in your workout with less intensity, mimicking the movement patterns, e.g, performing a bodyweight squat before performing a weighted squat in the workout. But for now, let's keep it simple!

Preparation

Start with 10 deep cleansing breaths to fill your lungs and muscles with oxygen. Breathe in deeply through your nose for 4-6 seconds or as long as you can, hold that breath for 1-2 seconds before slowly breathing out through your mouth for 4-6 seconds. Whilst you're taking these breaths, picture your body energizing, because it really is; in fact, breathing through your nose can allow you to take in up to 20% more oxygen than mouth breathing! With each breath, feel your energy increasing and your focus improving before being ready for the next challenge.

On the next page you'll find some different warmups you can try depending on your capabilities, so please pick the one most suitable for you.

Mobility Whilst Supine Lying

Supine means lying on your back and is great for those who have difficulty standing or sitting or would like to complete the mobility session before getting out of bed. Start with your legs flat or bent at the knee with your feet on the surface you're lying on, and after your cleansing breaths, perform the following sequence of movements:

1. **Neck Turns** - Allow your head to naturally fall to the right as if looking over your shoulder. Gently bring it back to the middle before allowing it to fall to the left. Perform this up to 10 times each side.

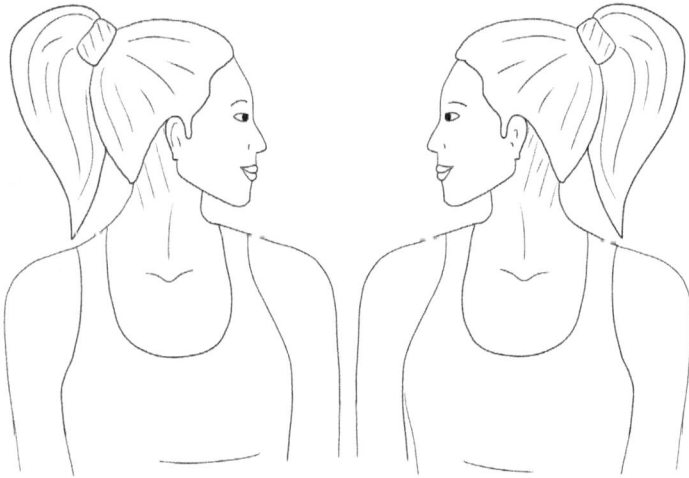

2. **Shoulder Rolls** - Allow your shoulders to roll forwards, then upwards towards the ears, then backwards whilst you squeeze your shoulder blades together, before returning to the starting point. Perform this up to 20 times, changing directions if you wish!

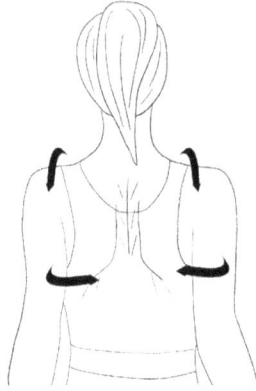

3. **Wrist Rolls** – Rotate the wrist 5 times to the right and 5 times to the left in a smooth action.

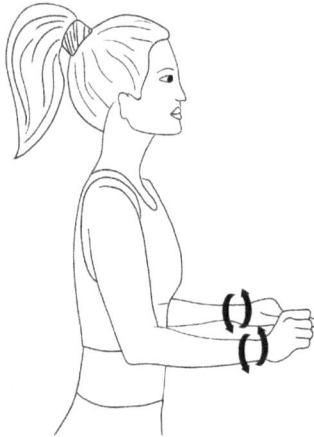

4. **Hand Openings** – Open the hands and fingers and stretch them out, then curl the fingers into a ball, squeezing the hands together. Perform this up to 20 times.

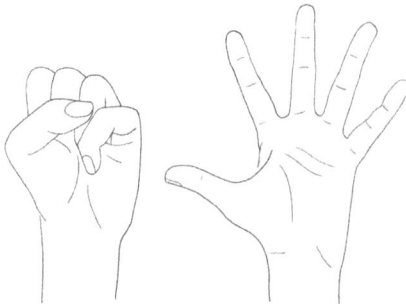

5. **Arm Slides** – Starting with your hands by your side, slide them upwards in a semi circle motion until they are parallel with the shoulders, as if making a cross with your arms and body. Slide your arms back to the starting point and repeat up to 10 times or more if you'd like a challenge.

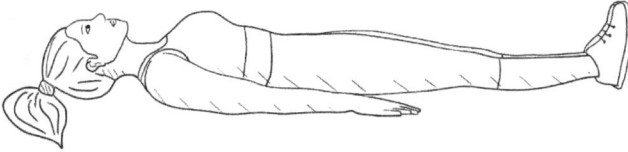

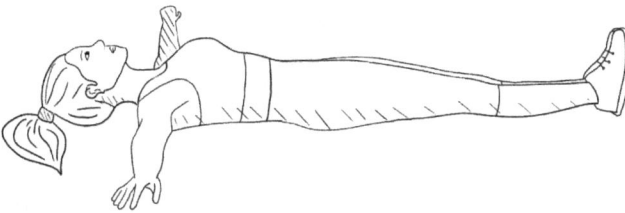

6. **Single Leg Slides** – Starting with both knees bent and your feet flat on your bed or other flat surface, slide one foot away from the body until the leg is straight, maintaining contact with the surface with the heel of the foot. Slide the foot back to the starting position and repeat on the other leg. Perform this up to 10 times on each leg.

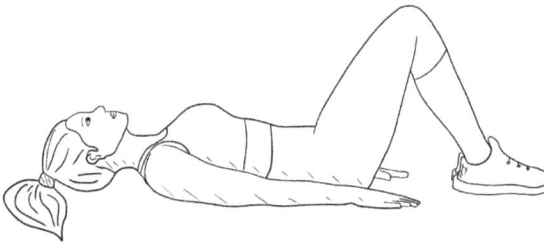

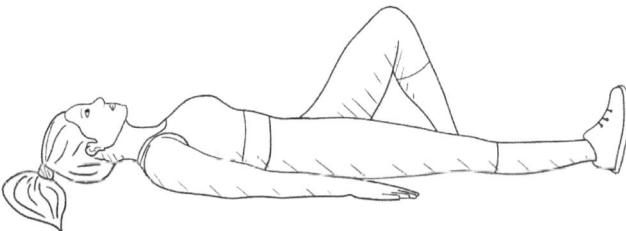

7. **Ankle Rolls** – Slide the leg away from the body as above, but this time leave the leg in the straight position, and roll the ankle five times to the right and five times to the left, completing full circles with the ankle. Draw the foot back to the starting position and repeat with the opposite leg. Repeat 10 times on each ankle.

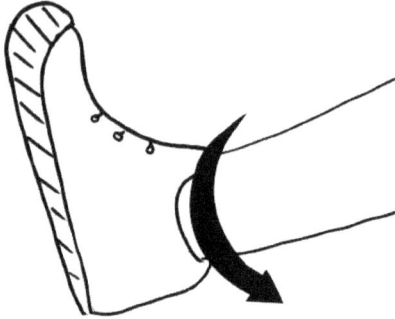

8. **10 and 2 Toes** – Start by lying with the legs straight and the toes facing upwards to 12 o'clock. Gently rotate at the hip and bring the left toes to a 10 o'clock angle and the right toes to a 2 o'clock angle, then return both feet back to 12 o'clock. If you are able to do so, then bring the toes inwards so the right foot is crossing the left at 10 o'clock and the left is crossing the right at 2 o'clock. Perform this up to 20 times.

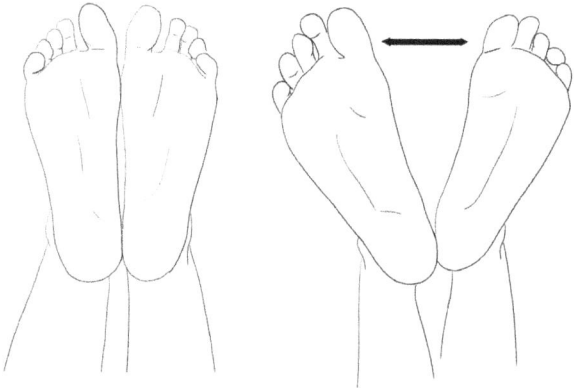

Now move on to your workout, which you can find from page 48 onwards!

Mobility Whilst Seated or Standing

Being in a seated or standing position can have a positive effect by adding a small amount of resistance to each movement. This can help with muscle strength and endurance, and postural care. Start in a comfortable seated or standing position; if you feel fatigued when standing, simply adopt a seated position and continue if you can. After your cleansing breaths, complete the following sequence of movements:

1. **Neck Turns** – Turn your head to the right as if looking over your shoulder, return to the start and turn your head to the left again as if looking over your other shoulder. Perform this up to 10 times in each direction.

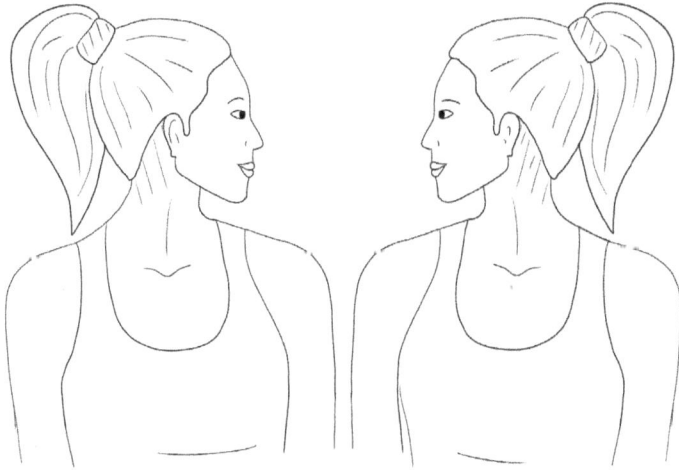

Whilst warming the neck muscles, you can also move your head up and down, allowing the head to fall under control as if placing your chin on your chest, then lift the head back to the starting position and gently lift the head as if looking at the ceiling. Don't lift too far so as to hurt the base of the neck. Return to the starting position and repeat up to 10 times. Gentle full neck rolls to finish are also great!

2. **Shoulder Rolls** – Allow your shoulders to roll forwards, then back upwards towards the ears, then backwards whilst you squeeze your shoulder blades together, before returning to the starting point. Perform this up to 20 times, changing directions if you wish!

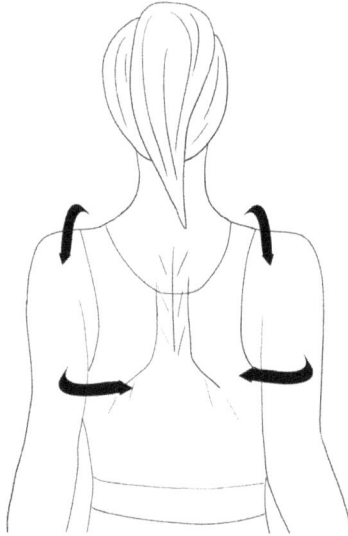

3. **Wrist Rolls** – Rotate the wrists 5 times to the right and 5 times to the right in a smooth action.

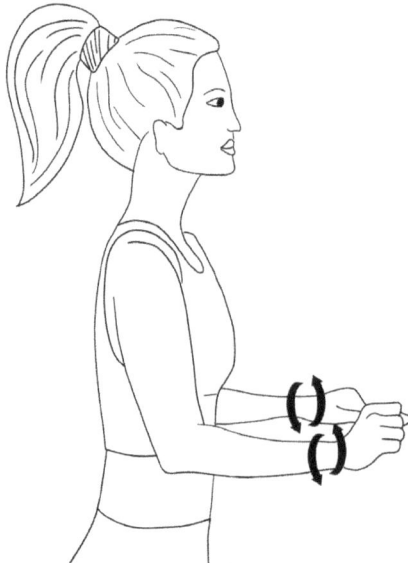

4. **Hand Openings** – Open the hands and fingers and stretch them out, then curl the fingers into a ball squeezing the hands together. Repeat up to 20 times.

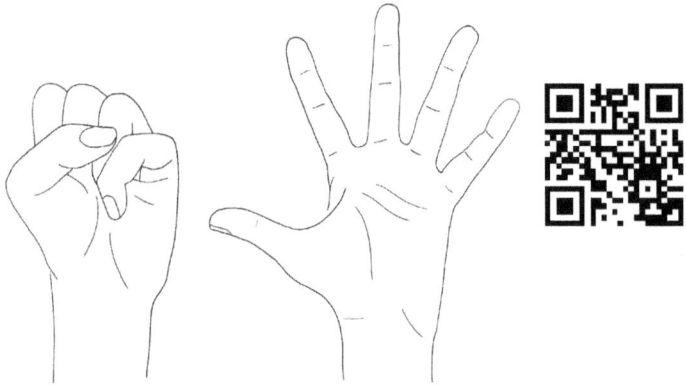

5. **Trunk Rotation** – Cross the arms across the chest with the elbows resting on the body, then gently twist the body allowing the trunk to rotate to one side, do not rotate too far so as to hurt the hips or lower back. Return to the start then rotate the opposite way. Perform this up to 10 times in each direction.

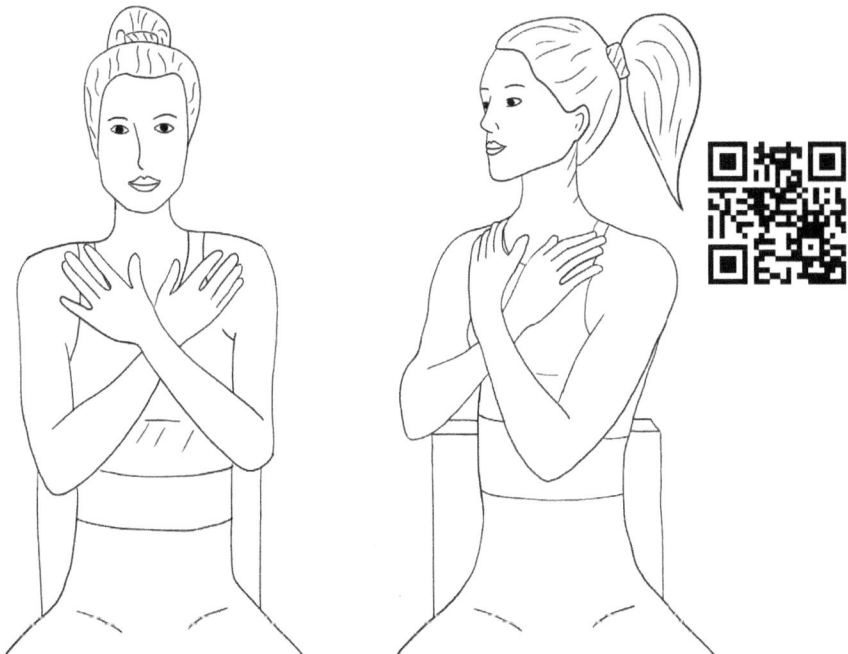

6. **Seated Leg Slides** – Starting in a seated position with both feet on the floor, slide one foot away from the body without lifting it off the ground. Slide that foot back to the starting position and repeat on the opposite side. Perform this up to 10 times with each leg.

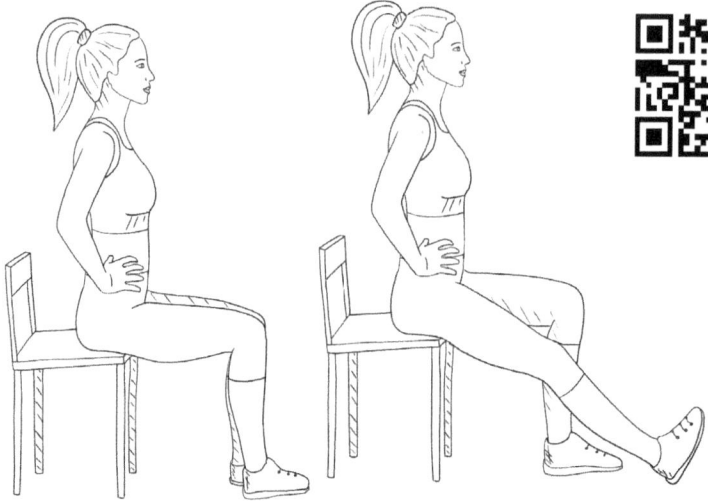

7. **Seated Heel-Toes** – Using a heel toe motion, walk one foot at a time out sideways using 6-8 small steps before walking it back in again. Repeat on the opposite leg. Perform this up to 10 times on each foot. If performing this movement whilst standing, hold onto a stable surface for support.

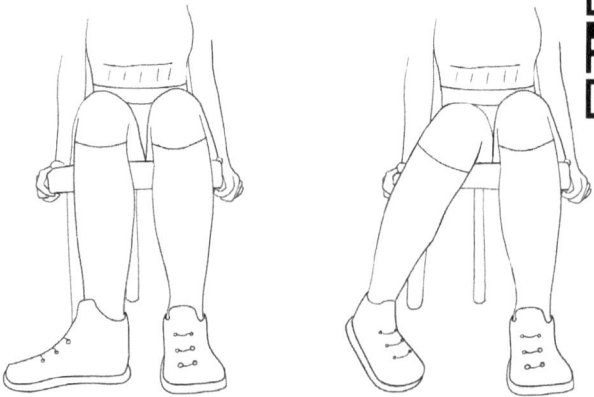

8. **Ankle Rolls** – Starting in a seated or standing position, slide one leg away from the body, extending it out to the front of you. Hold your leg in this extended position whilst rolling the ankle 5 times to the right and 5 times to the left completing full circles. Draw the foot back in and place it on the floor and repeat with the opposite leg.

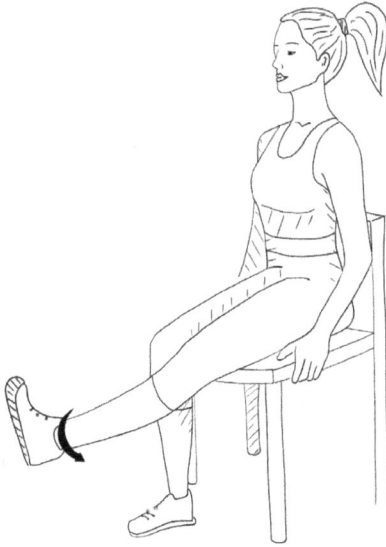

Now move onto your workout, which you can find from page 48 onwards!

Part 2. Chapter 6.

LET'S GET STRONG! (STRENGTH TRAINING PROGRAM AND PROGRESSIONS)

N ow that you're warm, it's time to get into your workout!

The following strength training programs have been developed to help you to improve your general strength, balance and mobility. But that's not all, sticking to your chosen plan long term can boost your energy, reduce your risk of falling, give you less aches and pains and help you to stay independent and active. Though these routines may seem simple to some, they can be very effective at helping you with a lot of the ailments that you may have come here to improve, so please trust the process and stay consistent with your new exercise routine until you see and feel improvements!

This plan has been created especially for you by a military Exercise Rehabilitation Instructor with over 15 years experience of helping people just like you. So I'll let him take it from here for the rest of this chapter!

Terminology you'll need to know for this section:

Reps = Repetitions. The number of times you perform a movement.

Set = The number of times you perform a certain number of repetitions, e.g, 3 sets of 10 reps.

Hello, Chris here! When embarking on any exercise program it is essential that you gradually progress the program from time to time. Every 3-4 weeks is suggested but this can differ from person to person. By progressing the program you are ensuring that you continue to maintain your current function or improve on your current function. When the exercise you are completing starts to become much easier or no longer challenging, that's a great time to progress. One to two small changes can make all the difference and it doesn't have to be on every exercise.

In the exercise programs to follow the exercises can be interchanged depending on your current level of function or your need to progress your program.

There are many ways to progress, here a few methods I usually suggest to my clients:

1. Perform more repetitions or sets of the same exercise than you previously did in your last workout. Each exercise listed in the program to follow comes with a suggested number of reps, so for a challenge you could add to those reps, or you could add a whole other set, or even perform the whole routine two or three more times in a row, rather than just once through.

2. Workout more frequently. Whilst you're starting your strength training journey even just two workouts per week will be a great start in terms of building your muscles and improving your balance and stability (amongst other benefits). But once your body is used to some more movement, adding in some more workouts throughout the week will allow you to reap even more benefits. We suggest working up to performing your exercise routine up to every other day. Rest and recovery is extremely important so this will still allow some time for your body to heal in between sessions

3. Perform a harder version of the exercise you are doing if progressions are suggested in the program. E.g, Try a movement standing up rather than sitting down to add the challenge of

balance/using more core strength. Or try a bodyweight squat rather than a sit-to-stand for example.

4. Add external resistance such as dumbbells or readily accessible objects like cans of beans or small water bottles to add a challenge to the movement.

The first step in your strength training journey, is to pick the level from the options below that you feel best suited to as a starting point:

1. **Level One:** Someone with a restricted lifestyle (limited function).

2. **Level Two:** Someone who is sedentary but able bodied to moderately active.

3. **Level Three:** Someone who is active.

You should perform the sequence of exercises listed at your chosen level initially over a 12 week period, on 2 to 4 days each week, adding progression through one of the methods listed above every 3-4 weeks or when you feel able. Once you have progressed within your chosen program after the suggested 12 weeks or whenever you feel ready for a new challenge, you can move to the next level up to continue progressing if able. I would recommend using a notebook to keep a record of how many repetitions and sets you perform of each exercise, as well as any weight you use, so that you're ensuring you're progressing week by week.

12 weeks is a motivational and realistic time frame to see real progression with strength, balance, energy, muscle tone and more, but the aim is that strength training becomes part of your life long term. Though we suggest you keep your exercise plan simple, so as to keep it effective and safe, once you feel comfortable with the movements in the following plan you can start adding movements from the exercise glossary into your workouts to add some variety and challenge. You can find this in Part 2, Chapter 8.

Please also remember to cool down and stretch after whatever workout you choose. You can find information on how to do this properly in Part 2, Chapter 7.

LEVEL 1: EXERCISE PROGRAM FOR PEOPLE WITH RESTRICTED LIFESTYLES

1. **Box Breathing**

   This exercise progressively challenges the major trunk muscles, there are three parts that form the box when carrying out the following steps:
   - **Step 1:** Sit or lie in a comfortable position with good posture (shoulders drawn together, chest up), gently draw the belly button inwards and hold whilst breathing normally. This forms two parts of the box as the muscles around the trunk wrap from front to back.
   - **Step 2:** Gently squeeze the glute muscles to form the bottom of the box. At this point by gently squeezing the undercarriage as if trying to stop yourself from peeing, you should be engaging the pelvic floor.
   - **Step 3:** Take long slow breaths and imagine the lungs filling sideways rather than forwards and backwards. This engages the diaphragm, a muscle essential for the breathing mechanism. Breathe in for around 4 seconds, hold for 1 and release for around 4 seconds. Repeat up to 10 times.

2. **Horizontal Row**

   In a seated or lying position push the arms out in front of you until they are straight and in line with the shoulders.

   Next, draw the arms back so the hands are at your side at chest height. Squeeze the shoulder blades together and hold for one second before repeating. If lying down, keep the hands in line with the bent elbows as the elbows and back of the upper arms touch the bed/surface.

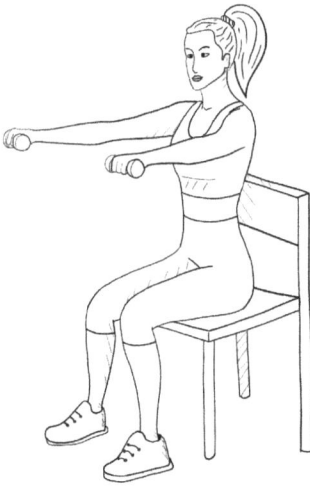

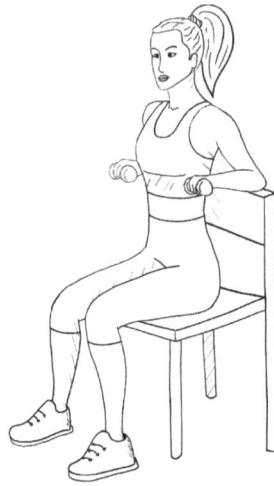

Perform this up to 12 times for a maximum of 3 sets.

3. **Seated Heel-Toe Raise**

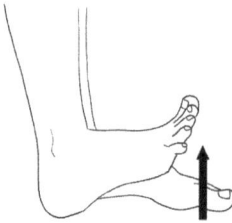

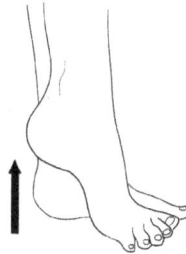

In a seated position with your feet flat on the floor, start by raising the toes of one foot off the ground as high as you are able to, then return to the ground.

On the same leg, then raise the heels off the ground as far as you are able to.

Swap feet and repeat!

Perform up to 10 times on each foot or perform with both feet at once for your chosen number of reps.

If unable to sit up, perform the same movement of moving your toes upwards, then pointing them down without the resistance of the floor whilst lying down.

4. Seated March

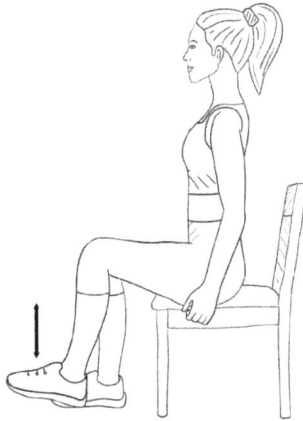

In a seated position with your feet flat on the floor, raise one leg off the ground by a few inches and slowly lower it back down. Change legs and repeat up to 20 times.

If unable to sit up, perform lying knee hugs instead, by lifting one bent leg towards your chest at a time and hugging it with your arms for up to 5 seconds before placing it back down straight and repeating with the other leg.

5. Wrist Rolls

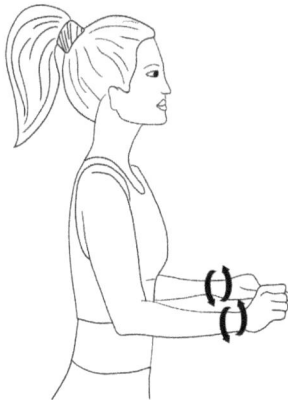

Bend your elbows to 90 degrees and slowly roll the wrists 5 times to the right and 5 times to the left.

Repeat this 5 times whilst taking 5 deep breaths and exhales.

6. Arm Curl and Overhead Press

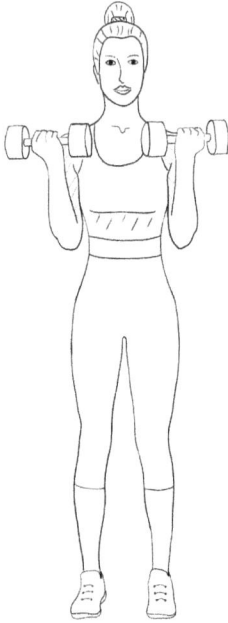

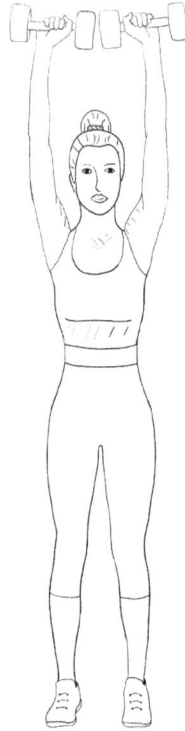

Sit on a stable chair if you can't stand to perform this exercise. Hold a dumbbell or household object like a bean can in each hand and bend your elbows so the hands are in line with the front of the shoulders, with the back of the hands facing away from the body (this is the arm curl).

Then rotate the hands so the palms are facing away from the body as you raise the arms up over the head. If the overhead lift is too hard, start with the curl and progress to both once you can. Perform for 3 sets of 10 if you can, with 20 resting breaths in between each set.

If you can't sit up, perform the arm curl as normal lying down, then press the weights up above your body rather than above your head.

7. Seated Leg Extension

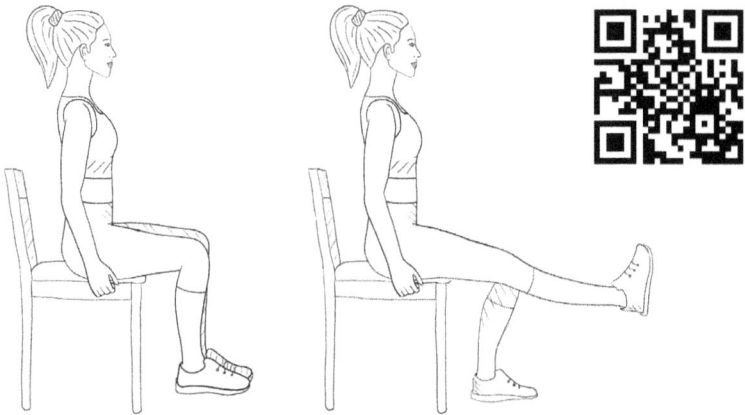

In a seated position with both feet placed on the ground, keep one foot on the ground whilst you straighten the other leg by contracting the thigh muscle.

Hold in the extended position for 5 seconds before lowering it slowly under control. Repeat on the other leg and perform up to 12 times on each leg.

If you can't sit up, lie on your bed with your knees in line with the edge of the bed and legs bent over the side and repeat the above instructions in this lying position instead!

8. Seated Leg Curls

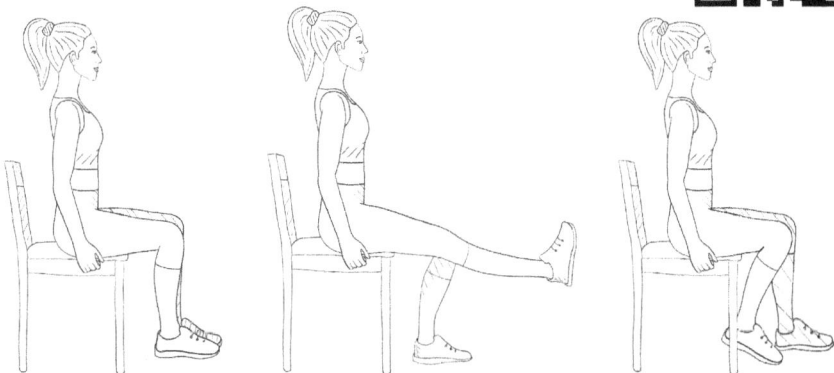

Sit on the edge of a bed or chair with one foot placed on the ground for support and one leg extended with the knee straight (like you just did for the leg extension).

Whilst bending the knee of the extended leg, pull the heel under the chair or bed frame by contracting the muscle on the back of the thigh. Hold for 5 seconds before relaxing slowly and placing the foot back on the floor.

Repeat on the other leg and perform up to 12 alternate leg curls.

Remember to progress this plan you could repeat the whole sequence after a 2-3 minute rest, or add weight to the movements, or repeat more sets of certain movements!

Now move on to your cool down, which you can find from page 83 onwards!

LEVEL 2: EXERCISE PROGRAM FOR PEOPLE WITH SEDENTARY TO MODERATELY ACTIVE LIFESTYLES

1. **Supported Small Glute Kickback**

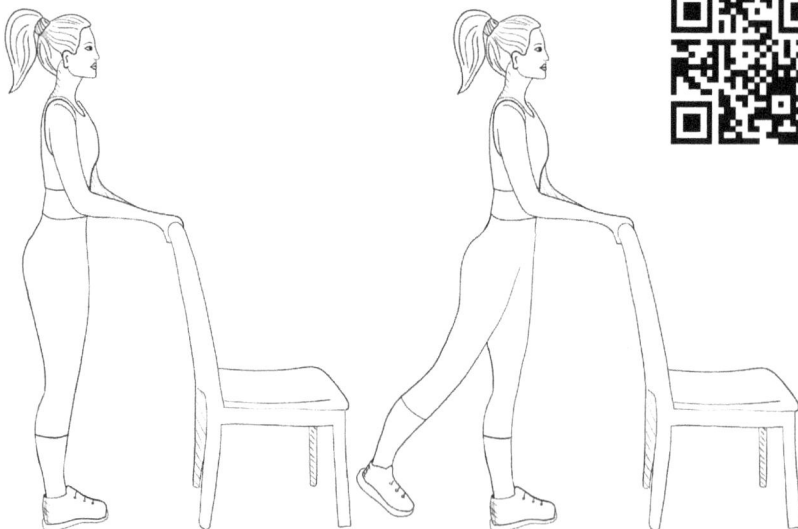

Use a raised firm surface as support throughout. Place both hands on the surface, with your feet shoulder width apart.

Perform a small knee bend on one leg whilst pushing the leg backwards slightly to engage the glute muscles. The range of movement depends on your own limitations but aim for up to 45 degrees or about 6-10cm of movement. Perform this movement with your upper body standing tall and your belly button pulled gently into the back.

Perform this up to 10 times on each leg with a 2 second hold. Repeat for more sets if desired!

2. Seated Calf Raise

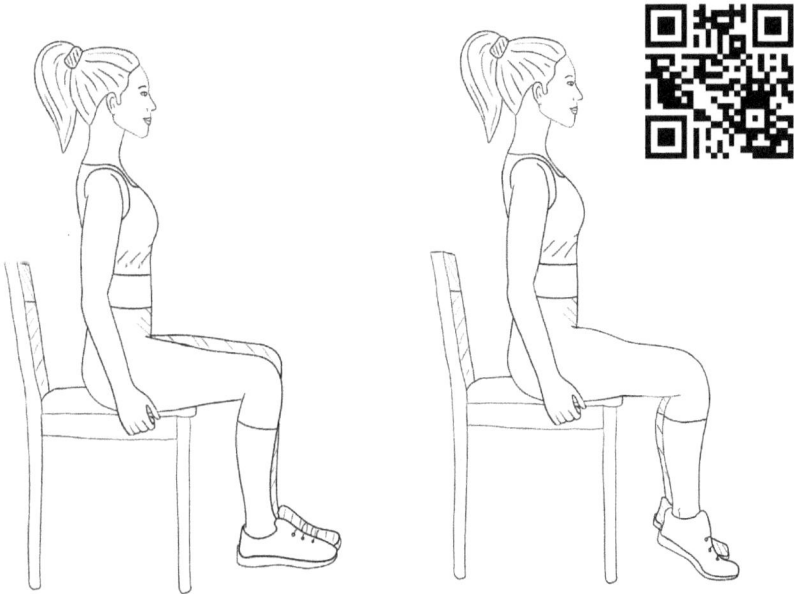

Find a comfortable seated position with your feet flat on the floor. Place the hands on the knees or side of the chair and lean slightly forwards. Lift the heels off the ground as far as you can without lifting your feet off the ground. Hold for one second and slowly lower back to the starting position.

Perform this up to 10 times for up to three sets.

3. Supported Single Leg Lift

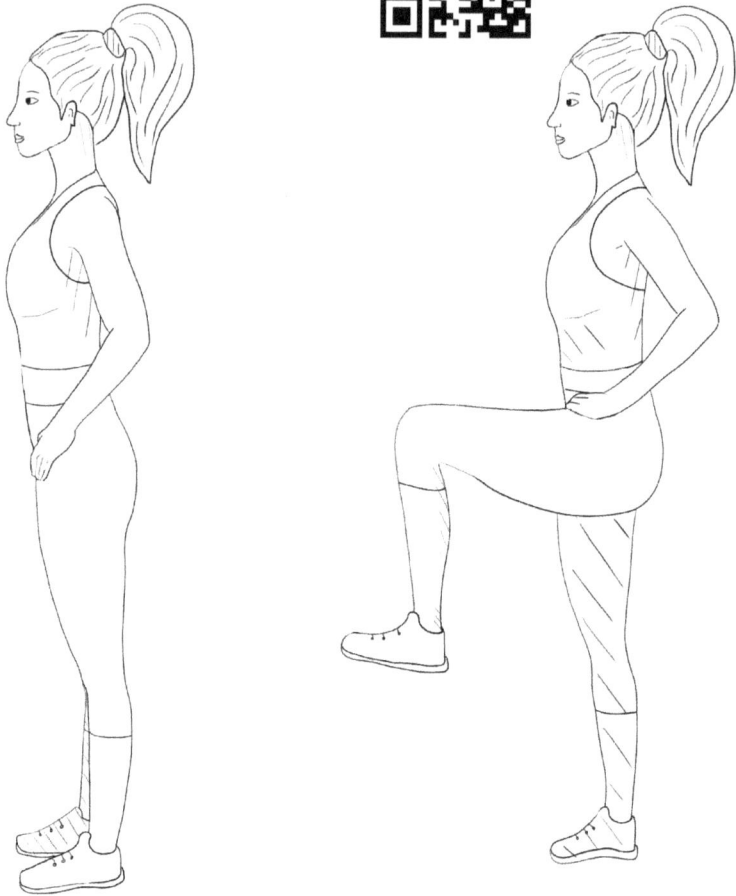

Place both hands on a raised support surface (or if you feel confident enough to balance, place your hands on your hips). Stand with your feet shoulder width apart and lift one leg off the floor, raising the knee towards the chest, only go as far as the thigh being parallel to the floor, pause for one second and slowly return to the starting position.

Change legs and repeat, perform up to 10 times on each leg. Take a 1-3 minute rest then repeat another 10 times on each leg.

4. Wall Angels

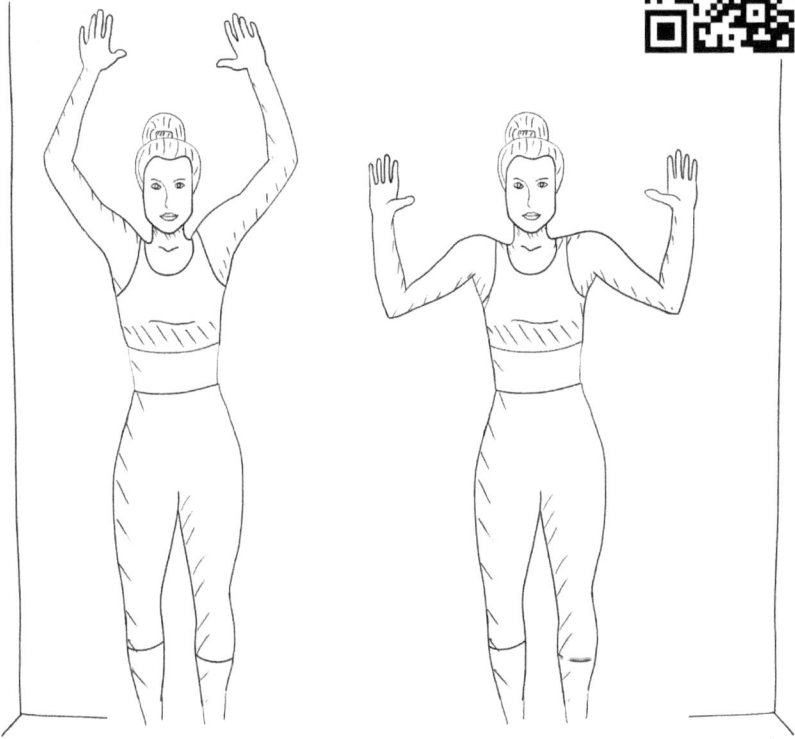

Find space on a wall and place your back against it with your shoulder blades and head in contact with the wall. Slowly place the arms out to either side of your body with a bend at the elbow, maintaining contact with the wall at all times.

Then raise the hands above the head as far as you feel comfortable, aiming for full range so the hands touch each other above the head.

Slowly return the arms back to the side of the body and repeat up to 10 times. Take a 1-2 minute rest then repeat!

5. Arm Curl and Overhead Press

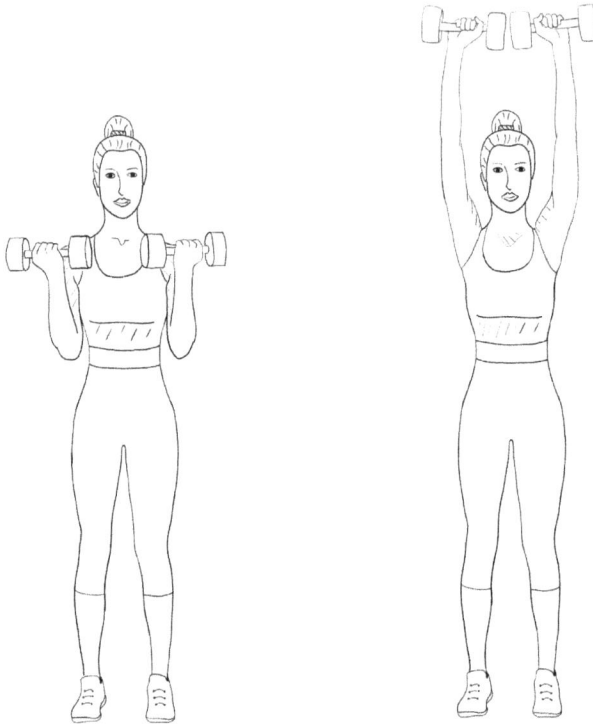

Stand with your feet shoulder width apart. Hold a dumbbell or household object like a bean can in each hand and bend your elbows so the hands are in line with the front of the shoulders, with the back of the hands facing away from the body (this is the arm curl).

Then rotate the hands so the palms are facing away from the body as you raise the arms up over the head. If the overhead lift is too hard, start with the curl and progress to both once you can.

Perform up to 3 sets of 10 if you can, with a 1-2 minute rest in between each set.

6. Glute Bridge

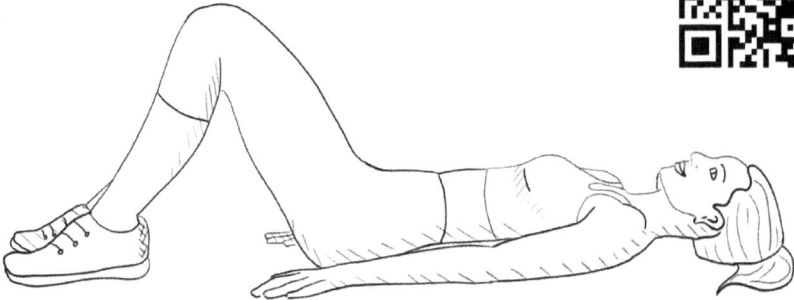

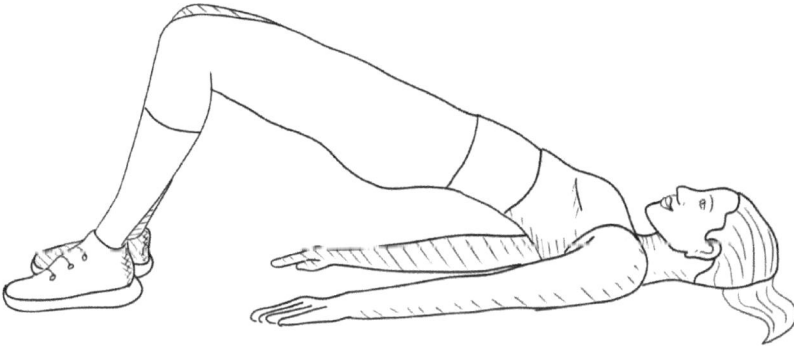

Lie on the floor with your knees bent and your feet flat on the floor, hands should be placed on the floor with the abs gently engaged by imagining pulling the belly button in towards the back. Squeeze the glute muscles as you lift the hips and torso off the floor, raising up as high as you can, trying to finish with thighs and torso in a diagonal line.

Slowly lower under control and repeat. Perform for 3 sets of 10 if you can, with a 1-2 minute rest in between each set.

7. Four Point Shoulder Taps

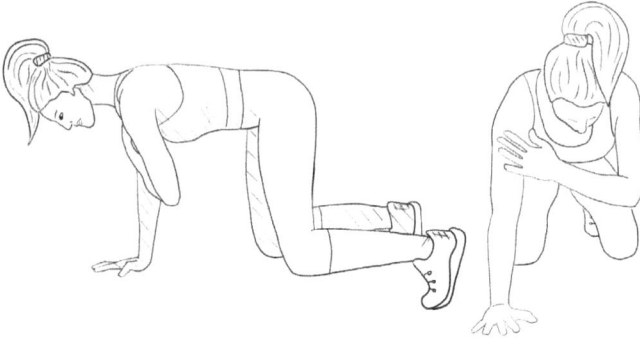

This exercise starts in the four point kneeling position: Kneeling on the floor with hands below the shoulders and knees below the hips, creating a table top position with the back. Use a mat or soft rug to protect the knees if possible.

Imagine drawing the belly button gently into the back whilst squeezing the glute muscles. Raise one hand and touch the opposite shoulder, then place it back on the floor and repeat with the other hand on the other shoulder. Perform this up to 12 times on each side.

Rest for 1-2 minutes and repeat!

8. Shopping Bag Hold

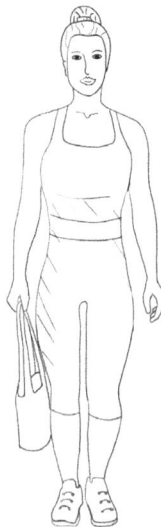

Grab a strong shopping bag with a short handle and place 2-3 items in the bag weighing a total of between 2-4kg. With the legs shoulder width apart, hold the bag at your side in one hand. Maintain an upright posture and don't lean towards or away from the bag. Hold for 5-10 seconds whilst taking deep breaths before changing sides and repeating.

When you've built up a good level of strength, try a Shopping Bag Carry: Walking from one side of the room to the other holding the bag with your core braced and upright. You could also slowly increase the weight in the bag to add more resistance.

Remember to progress this plan you could repeat the whole sequence after a 2-3 minute rest, or add weight to the movements, or repeat more sets of certain movements!

Now move onto your cool down, which you can find from page 83 onwards!

LEVEL 3: EXERCISE PROGRAM FOR PEOPLE WITH AN ACTIVE AND ABLE LIFESTYLE

1. Sit to Stand

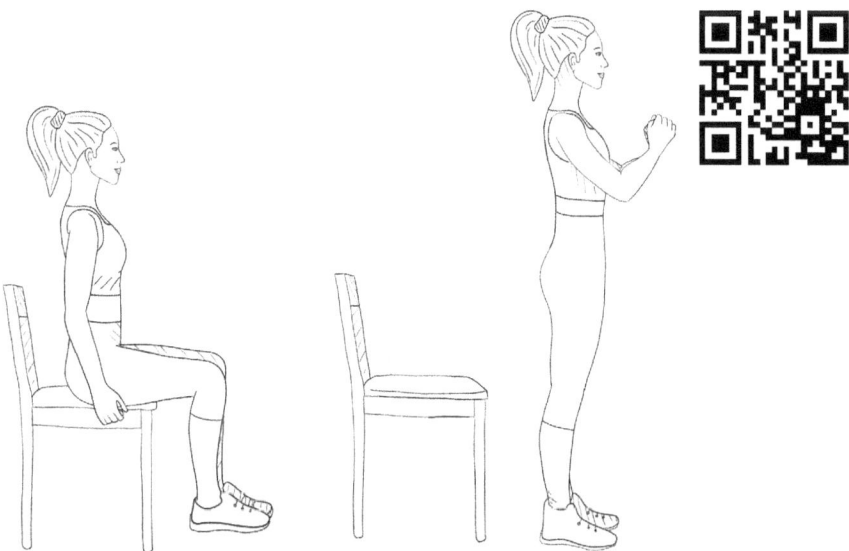

Use a sturdy chair for this exercise. This movement can be performed supported (using your hands to push you up off the chair) or unsupported. Engage the trunk muscles by drawing the belly button towards the back and squeezing the glute muscles.

With your feet placed apart, stand up in one motion before slowly supporting yourself back to a seated position. Use your arms to guide you down to the seat until confident. Repeat up to 10 times.

Perform up to 3 sets of 10 reps with a 1-2 minute rest inbetween sets.

2. **Supported Calf Raises**

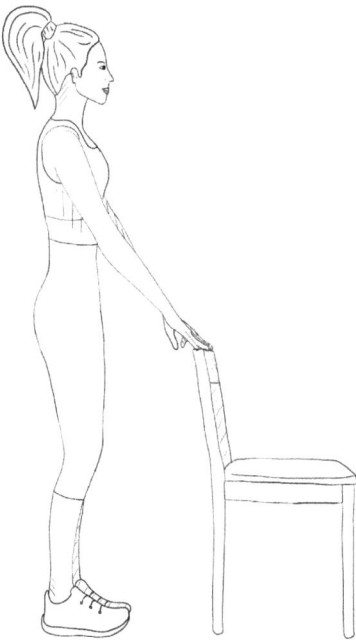

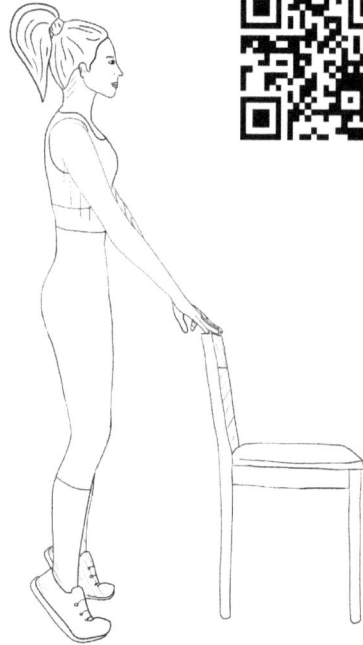

Place both hands on your support surface, with your feet shoulder width apart. Slowly raise both heels off the ground together as far as you feel comfortable to do so.

Pause for one second at the top of the movement before slowly lowering back to the start. Repeat up to 10 times.

Perform up to 3 sets of 10 reps with a 1-2 minute rest inbetween sets.

3. Standing Knee Lift and Tap

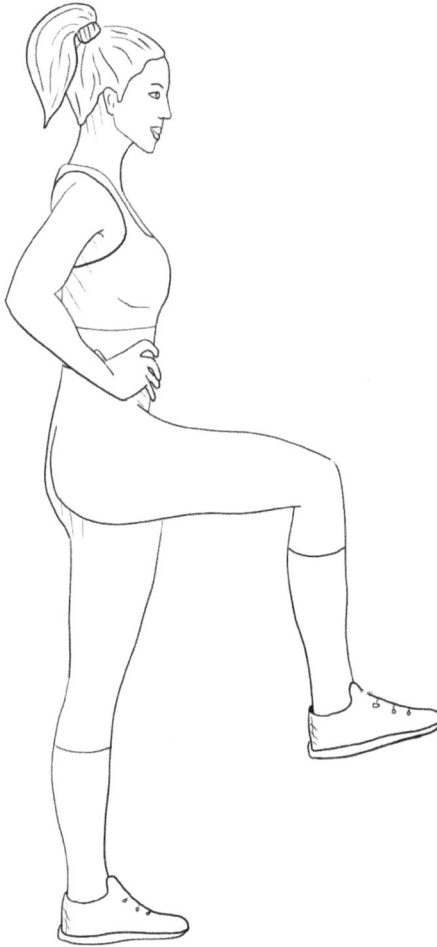

Standing with your feet shoulder width apart and your hands on your hips, raise one leg bringing the knee towards the chest until the thigh is parallel with the ground. Hold the leg for one second and touch the knee with the opposite hand.

Return the leg slowly under control and repeat on the opposite side. Repeat up to 10 times on each side.

Perform this for 2 or 3 more sets of 10 reps with a 1-2 minute rest inbetween sets.

4. Door Frame Trunk Rotations

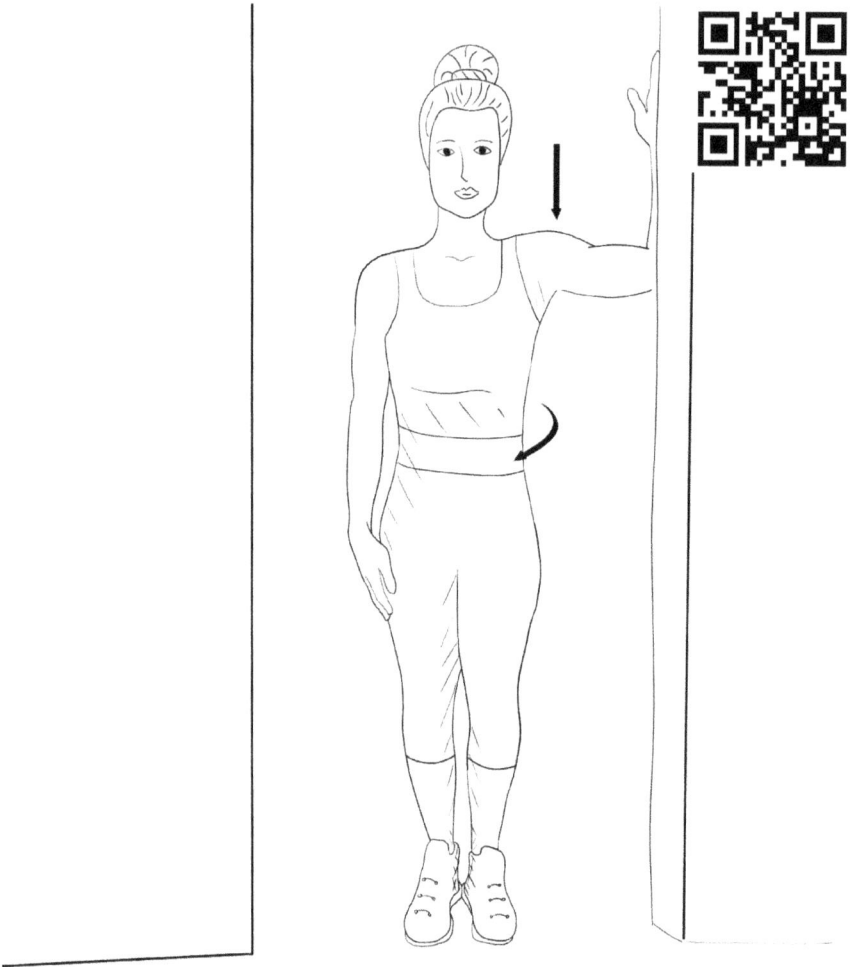

Stand with your feet naturally under the body inside a door frame. Place one hand out in front and against the door frame with the palm on the wall.

Press against the wall and you should feel several muscles starting to work such as the chest, the upper arm and trunk. The hip, glute and thigh muscles should also activate.

Hold for 5-10 seconds at about 50% of your maximum effort, change arms and repeat. Perform up to 2-4 times on each arm.

5. Wall Push Ups

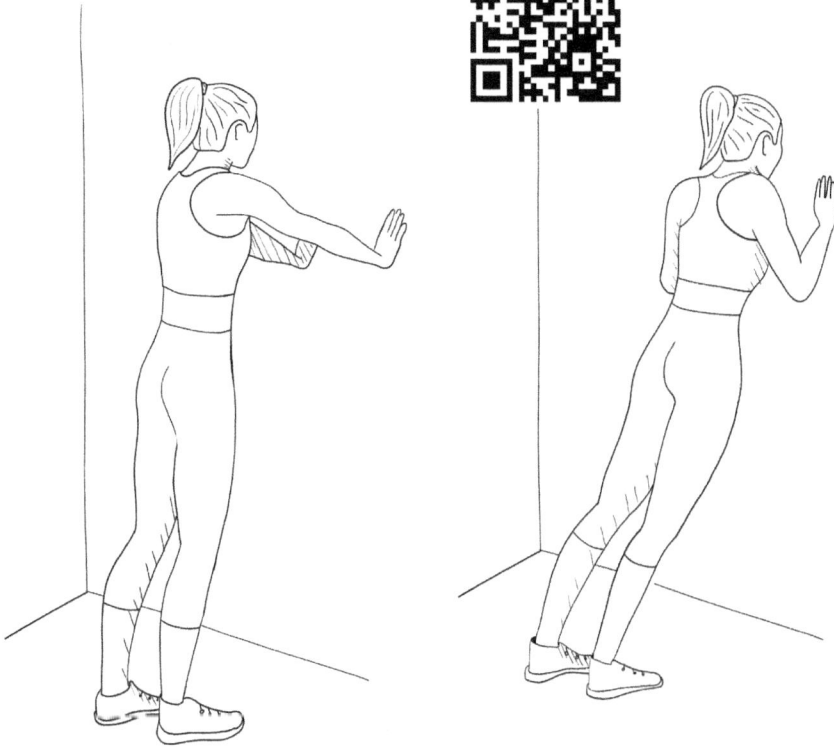

Place your hands shoulder width apart against a solid wall with your feet apart and weight naturally under the body. Bend at the elbows to bring the body towards the wall as far as you feel comfortable. Straighten the arms again to push away from the wall.

If you feel you can't lift your full weight, bring one foot forwards for assistance. If you'd like more of a challenge, try stepping a few steps away from the wall so that your push ups are being performed on a steeper angle, adding more resistance.

Repeat this up to 10 times for 3 sets with a 1-2 minute rest inbetween sets.

6. Glute Bridge

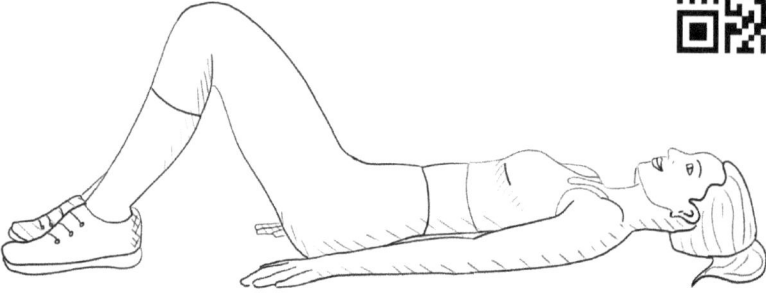

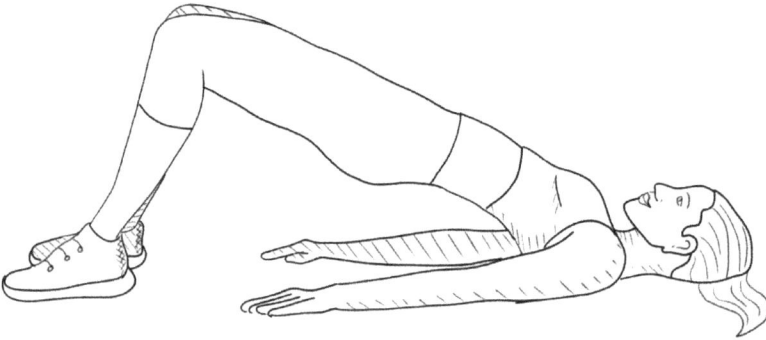

Lie on the floor with your knees bent and feet flat on the floor, hands should be placed on the floor with the abs gently engaged by imagining pulling the belly button in towards the back.

Squeeze the glute muscles as you lift the hips and torso off the floor, raising up as high as you can, trying to finish with your thighs and torso in a diagonal line. Slowly lower under control and repeat up to 10 times.

Perform for 3 sets of 10 reps if you can, with a 1-2 minute rest in between each set.

7. Dead Bugs

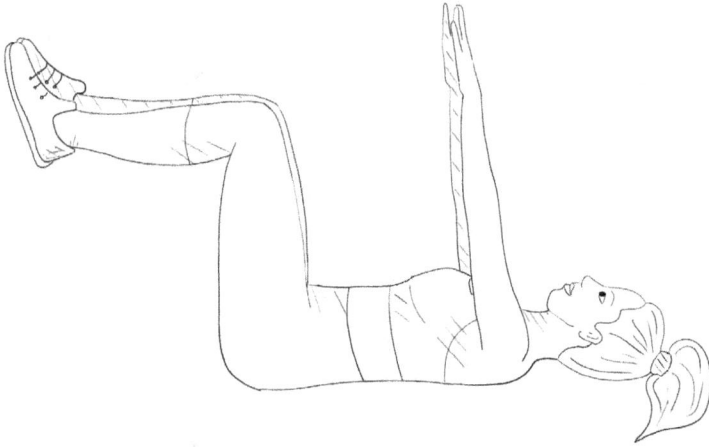

Lying on your back, lift the legs and bend the knees at a 90 degree angle with the shins parallel to the ground.

Raise the arms straight above the body to complete the starting position.

There are three progressions to try:

- **Progression 1:** Lower one leg or one arm at a time in the sequence of left leg, right leg, left arm, right arm. Keep the knees bent when lowering the legs and touch the ground with the toes, lower the arms above the head or to the side, whichever you feel more comfortable doing. Repeat up to 5 times on each limb for a total of 20 movements. After a short rest try a second or third set.

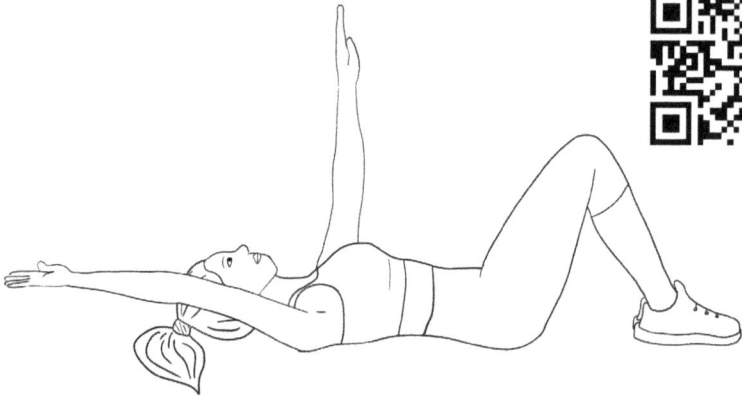

- **Progression 2:** Lower one leg to the floor with the knee staying bent whilst the supporting foot is on the floor. At the same time lower the opposite arm to the floor above the head or to the side of the body. Lift them both back to the starting position and repeat on the opposite side. Perform up to 10 times on alternating sides. After a short rest try a second or third set.

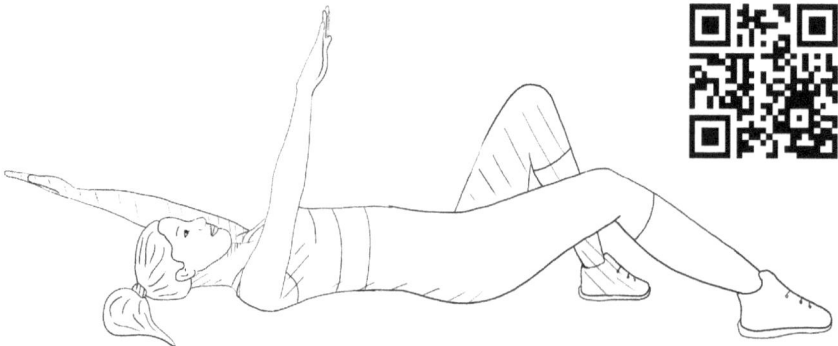

- **Progression 3:** Starting with both knees bent above the body, lower one leg to the floor, but this time straighten the leg so that it's parallel to the floor. At the same time lower the opposite arm to the floor above the head. Lift them both back to the starting position and repeat on the opposite side. Perform up to 10 times on alternating sides. After a short rest try a second or third set.

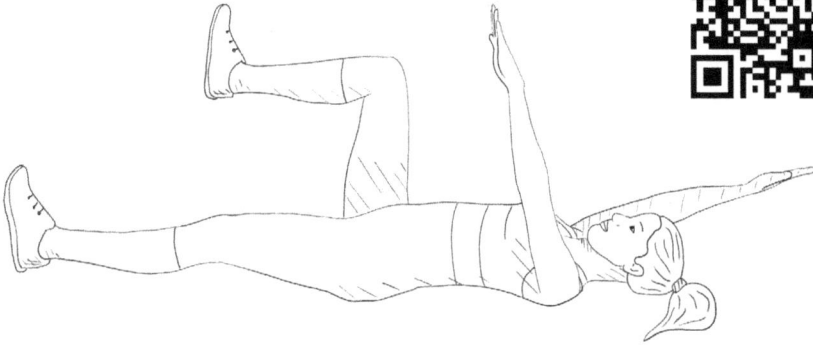

8. Superman Exercise

This exercise is an excellent all-rounder as it strengthens the core, leg and shoulder muscles and increases coordination. This exercise starts in the four point kneeling position - on the floor with hands below the shoulders and knees below hips, creating a table top position with the back. Use a mat or a soft rug to protect the knees. Perform 10 alternate movements of the progression of your choice, up to three times with a short rest in between each set.

There are 8 progressions to this exercise. Start with the most simple, then challenge yourself to try the next progression as soon as you feel able to!

- **Progression 1:** Shoulder Taps - In the four point kneeling position, raise one hand and touch the opposite shoulder, hold for one second and return to the starting position before repeating on the other side. Repeat for your desired number of reps.

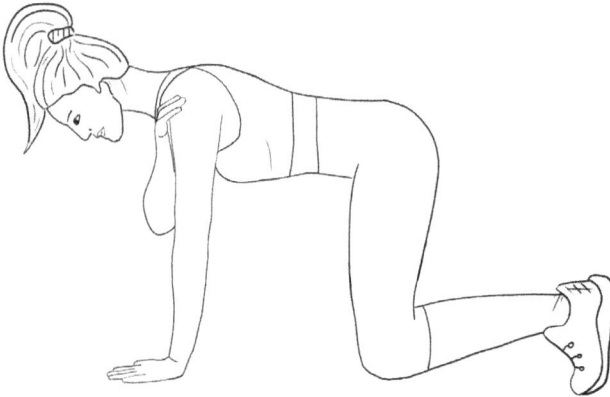

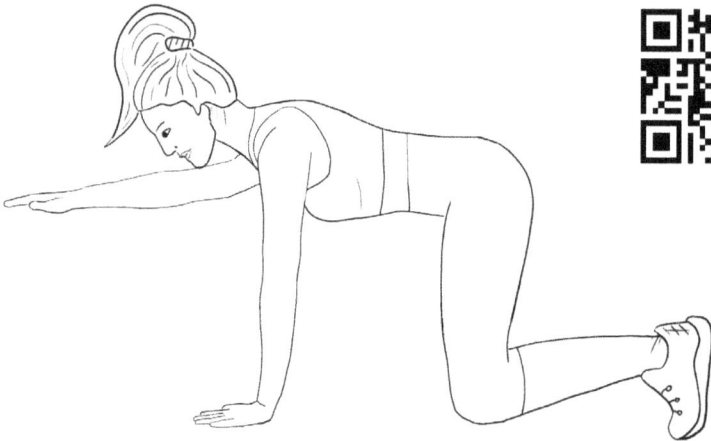

- **Progression 2:** Superman Arms - In four point kneeling, raise one arm straight out to the front in a superman position, hold for one second and return to the starting position before repeating on the other side. Repeat for your desired number of reps.

- **Progression 3:** Single Leg Slides - In four point kneeling, slide one leg backwards as far as is comfortable, keeping the toes on the floor. Stop when the leg is straight and do not lift the leg. Hold for one second and return to the starting position before repeating on the other side. Repeat for your desired number of reps.

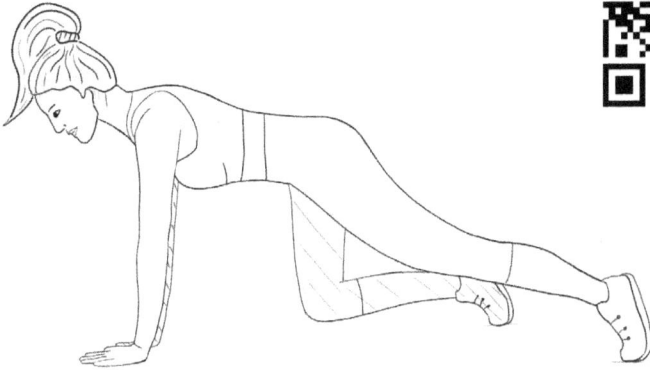

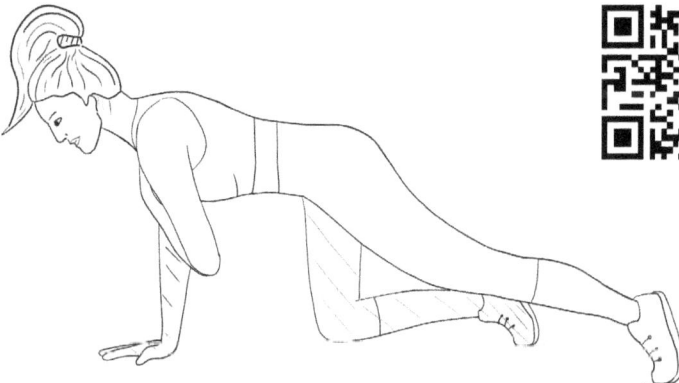

- **Progression 4:** Leg Slides and Shoulder Taps - In four point kneeling, slide one leg backwards as far as is comfortable, keeping the toes on the floor. Stop when the leg is straight and do not lift the leg. This time, add a one hand shoulder touch with the opposite arm than the leg that is pushed back. Hold for one second and return to the starting position before repeating on the other side. Repeat for your desired number of reps.

- **Progression 5:** Leg Slides and Superman Arms - In four point kneeling, slide one leg backwards as far as is comfortable, stop when the leg is straight but do not lift the leg off the floor. Perform a superman arm position with the opposite arm than the leg that is pushed back. Hold for one second and return to the starting position before repeating on the other side. Repeat for your desired number of reps.

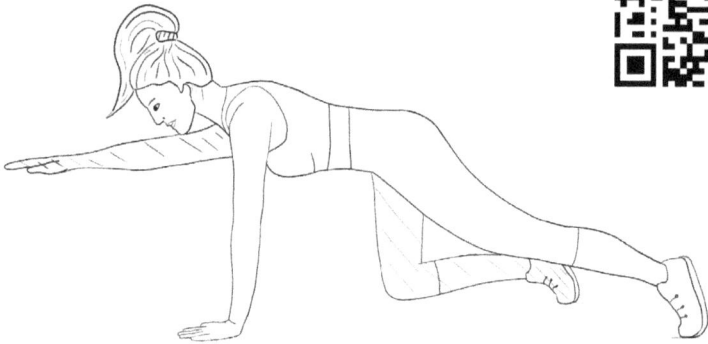

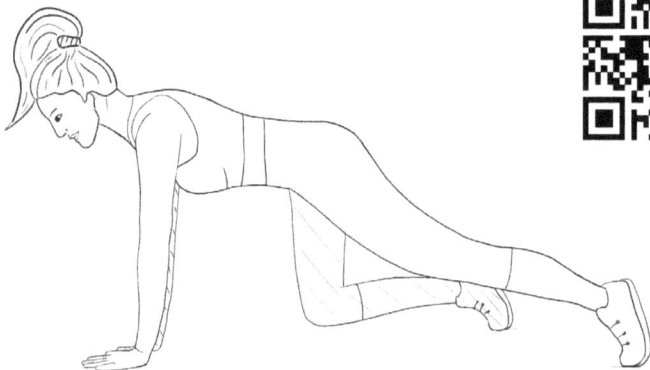

- **Progression 6:** Single Leg Lifts - In four point kneeling, slide one leg backwards as far as is comfortable, stop when the leg is straight and lift the leg slightly off the ground. Hold for one second and return to the starting position before repeating on the other side. Repeat for your desired number of reps.

- **Progression 7:** Single Leg Lifts and Shoulder Touches - In four point kneeling, slide one leg backwards as far as is comfortable, stop when the leg is straight and lift the leg slightly off the ground. This time add a one hand shoulder touch with the opposite arm than the leg that is performing the lift. Hold for one second and return to the starting position before repeating on the other side. Repeat for your desired number of reps.

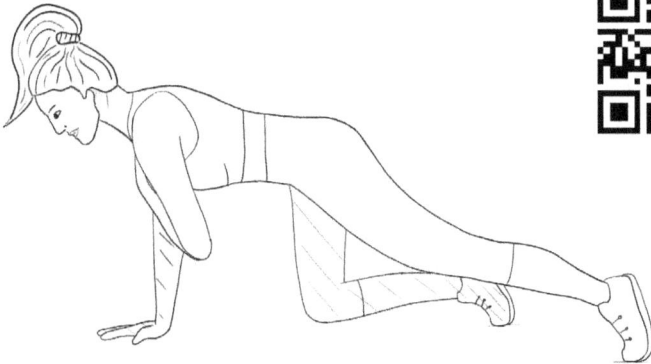

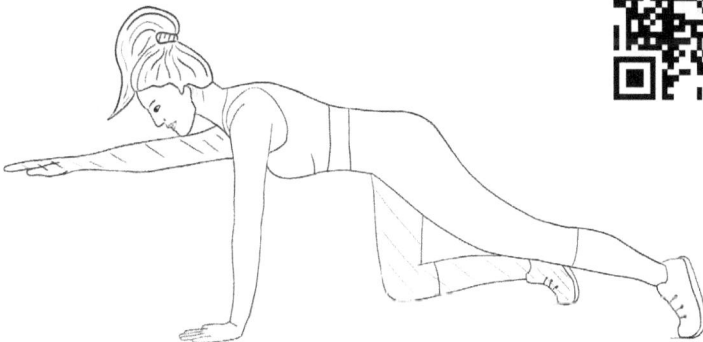

- **Progression 8:** Single Leg Lifts and Superman Arms - In four point kneeling, slide one leg backwards as far as is comfortable, stop when the leg is straight and lift the leg slightly off the ground. This time perform a superman arm position with the opposite arm than the leg that is pushed back. Hold for one second and return to the starting position before repeating on the other side. Repeat for your desired number of reps.

Remember to progress this plan you could repeat the whole sequence after a 2-3 minute rest, or add weight to the movements, or repeat more sets of certain movements!

Now move onto your cool down, which you can find from page 83 onwards!

Summary

For some, these exercises may seem difficult and unachievable, but I have no doubt that you are capable of doing these with some time and practice. Start with the most basic version of each exercise and you'll soon be surprising yourself with your progress. For others, these routines may seem simple, but when performed regularly (at least 3 times a week), they will improve your strength, balance and mobility (if you're fuelling your body properly, too!). Simple is often the best way forward, so trust the process and embrace the positive change coming to you!

I'd also advise writing down the sequence of your chosen workout plan so that once you've used the instructions, QR codes and illustrations to learn the movements, you can workout without having to flick through pages in between your exercises! If you'd like me to do this for you please email me at sophie@strongandstretchy.co.uk.

You're now on your way to reaping the benefits of strengthening your muscles and increasing your mobility and will soon find yourself looking for new ways to challenge yourself, mind, body and soul. My hope is that you surprise yourself with just how much strength and energy you can gain in a short amount of time!

I'd love to hear all about your results - please email me at sophie@strongandstretchy.co.uk with your story!

Please keep in mind that it is important to consult with your doctor before trying any new exercises or beginning a workout routine if you have health issues or are on medication.

Part 2. Chapter 7.

TIME TO CHILL!

So, how did you enjoy your strength training session? You're back with me, Sophie now, and I'm here to tell you some great news; you've done the hard work and it's now time to chill!

And by 'chill', I mean cool down and relax. A cool down is just as important as a good warm up. It will help your heart rate, body temperature, and blood pressure to return to their normal levels safely. Incorporating some gentle stretches into your cool down will also help to improve your flexibility and mobility and after a workout can help reduce the build-up of lactic acid, meaning there's less chance of muscle cramps and stiffness. Flip the page to see some staple stretches to try after your workout before you cooldown.

Cat-Cow

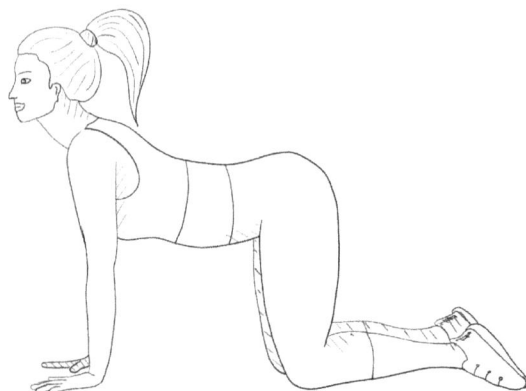

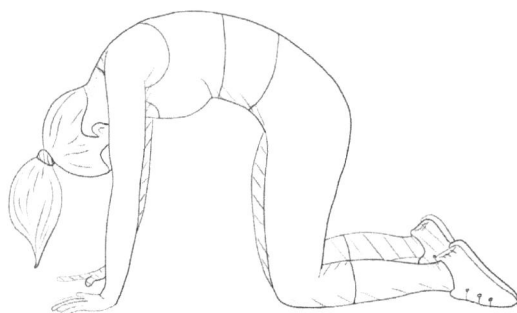

How to perform the Cat-Cow stretch:

- **Step 1 – Get into position:** Begin on all fours in the tabletop position with a neutral spine. Gently gaze forward.
- **Step 2 – Cow pose:** As you inhale, move into 'cow pose' by lifting your sit bones upward and pressing your chest forward. Allow your belly to sink and lift your head. Keep your shoulders relaxed and away from your ears. Keep your gaze straight ahead.
- **Step 3 – Cat pose:** As you exhale, move into 'cat pose' by rounding your spine outward and upward and tucking your tailbone under. Slowly draw your pubic bone forward and release your head toward the floor. There is no need to force your chin to your chest, keep your neck long.

- **Step 4 – Repeat:** Transition back into the 'cow' position and repeat as many times as needed. Most importantly, relax, enjoy and breathe.

Primary Muscles Stretched: The 'cat-cow' pose increases the flexibility of your neck, spine, and shoulders. This movement also stretches the hips, back, chest and abdomen.

Helps With: Releasing tension in the neck and back. It can also improve posture and when paired with some deep breaths, can be a very relaxing movement.

If you can't get into the tabletop position, you can do a variation of this movement sitting on a chair by creating the forwards and backwards curve motion in your spine

Child's Pose

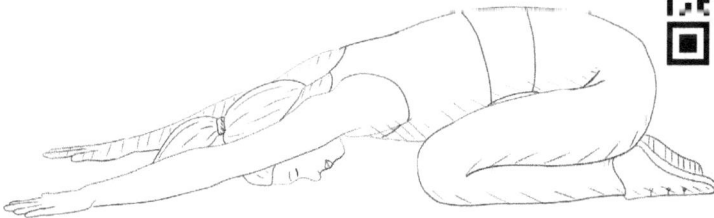

How to perform the Child's Pose stretch:
- **Step 1 – Get into position:** Kneel on your exercise mat or soft surface with your knees hip-width apart and your toes together. Rest your palms gently on your thighs and take a big deep breath.
- **Step 2 – Stretch forward:** On an exhale, lower your torso towards your knees and extend your arms forward with your palms facing down, pressed onto the mat/floor. Relax your shoulders toward the ground. Rest in this stretch for as long as needed and picture your aches and pains dissipating into the ground as you allow the floor to take your weight.

Primary Muscles Stretched: The child's pose stretches mainly the back muscles. If you have tight back and hip muscles, this pose may feel like work at first but take it slow and only go as far as is comfortable.

Helps With: Through relaxing into the position and breathing deeply, the childs pose can calm your mind and reduce stress and fatigue. It's great for releasing tension in your lower back, hamstrings, chest, and shoulders and can even provide relief for those with sciatica.

If you can't get into this position on the floor, you can do a variation of this movement sitting on a chair, by folding your upper body over your legs whilst sitting. Allow your arms to dangle down in front of you and picture all of the weight of your head dropping down onto the floor. Make sure you return to sitting upwards very slowly to avoid any dizziness.

Knees-to-Chest

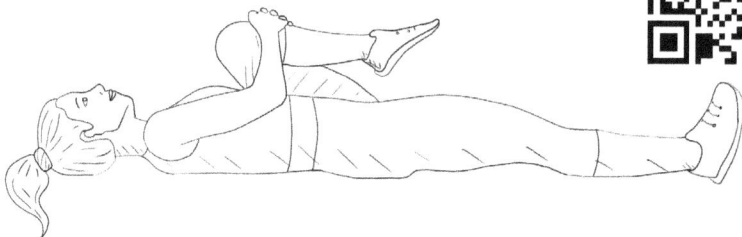

How to perform the Knees-to-Chest stretch:
- **Step 1 – Get into position:** Lie on your back on an exercise mat or bed with your feet a little over hip-width apart. Exhale and slowly bring one or both knees towards your chest.
- **Step 2 – Hug your knee/s:** Relax and soften your shoulders whilst allowing your head and body to sink into the mat/bed. Place your hands on your knee/s and hug your leg/s into your chest. Hold for as long as needed before resting and repeating or performing with the other leg if doing single knee-to-chest stretches.

If you can sit up you could also try a variation of this stretch in a chair:

- **Step 1 – Get into position**: Sit up straight on a supportive chair. Plant both feet on the ground.
- **Step 2 – Hug your knee:** Grasp the back of your right knee and slowly bring it towards your chest as far as is comfortable, whilst your left foot stays flat on the floor. Hold the position taking 2 deep breaths, then place the foot back on the floor and repeat with the other leg.

Primary Muscles Stretched: The knees-to-chest pose stretches mainly your hips, glutes, and lower back muscles. It can also help relieve pressure on your spinal nerves.

Helps With: Stabilizing your pelvis and lower back, and can help to reduce lower back pain.

Head Tilt with Resistance

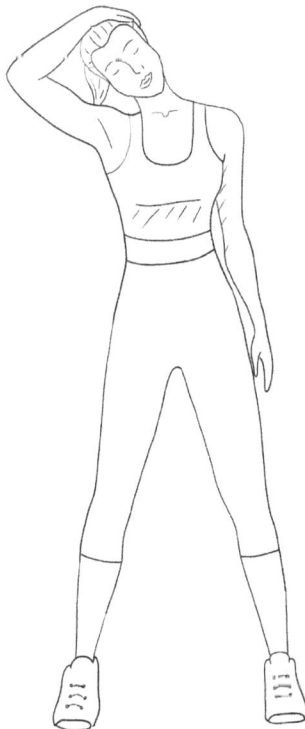

How to perform the Standing Head Tilt with resistance:

- **Step 1 – Get into position:** Begin by sitting upright on a sturdy chair or standing with your feet slightly wider than shoulder width apart.
- **Step 2 – Stretch:** First, bring your right ear towards your right shoulder. Take care not to bring your shoulder up, allow your head to fall towards it. Keep your shoulders relaxed. Use your right hand to gently provide some resistance to feel a deeper stretch on the side of the neck. Do not pull too hard. Take 5 deep breaths as you relax into the stretch, then slowly return the head to the center and repeat the stretch on the other side.

This stretch can also be performed lying down

Primary Muscles Stretched: The head tilt primarily stretches the muscles on both sides of your neck but also provides a nice stretch for the upper Trapezius.

Helps With: Improving and preserving the range of motion and elasticity of the neck, relieving the stiffness that often contributes to neck pain. Tight neck muscles can also cause headaches so this could even get rid of that pesky headache that's been getting you down!

Windshield Wiper

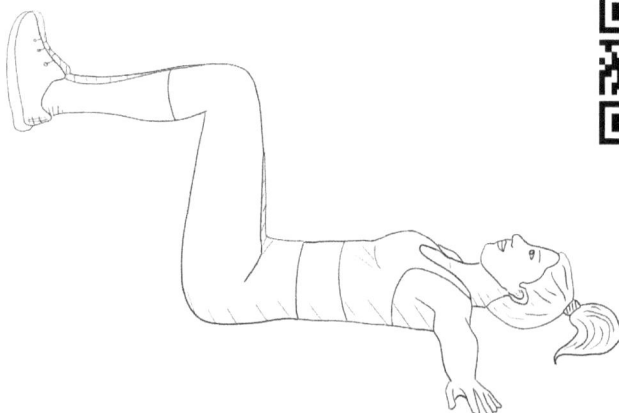

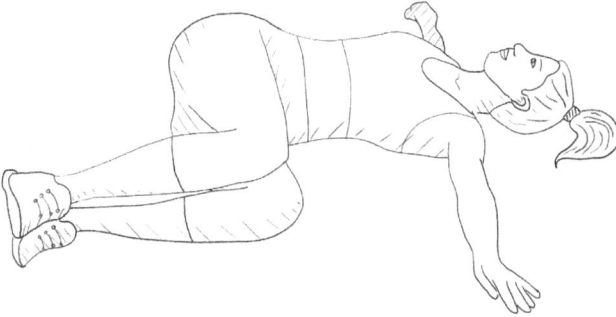

How to perform the Windshield Wiper movement:

- **Step 1 – Get into position:** Lie on your back on an exercise mat or soft surface with your arms out to the sides and your legs straight. Bend your knees to a 90-degree angle.

- **Step 2 – Wipe!:** Rotate your hips to one side, gently lowering your legs to the floor as if wiping a windshield. Hold this lowered position and take some deep breaths as you feel the stretch. Then, lift your legs and return to the starting position, keeping your knees bent. Rotate your hips to the opposite side and repeat. Be sure to keep your shoulders as flat on the floor as possible.

Primary Muscles Stretched: The 'windshield wiper' stretches mainly the obliques and abdominal muscles, as well as the back. It also activates the glutes and hip flexors, helping to strengthen those.

Helps With: Building a stronger core as well as providing a comforting stretch in the lower back which is great for relieving back pain. It also strengthens the lower back muscles and hip flexors which improves daily mobility.

Seated Figure 4 Glute Stretch

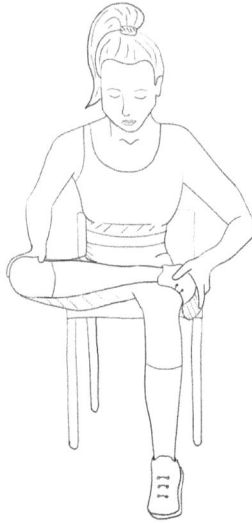

How to perform the Figure 4 Glute Stretch:

- **Step 1 – Get into position:** Sit on a chair and keep one foot placed on the ground.
- **Step 2 – Create the figure 4:** Place the outside of the other lower leg on the thigh of the supporting leg, creating a figure 4. If you can't bring the leg up into this position, cross the outside of the lower leg over the shin of your other leg.
- **Step 3 - Bend:** Slowly bend your torso over the legs, only as far as is comfortable. Hold this position for up to five seconds before placing the foot back on the floor, then repeat on the other side.

Primary Muscles Stretched: The glutes!

Helps With: Loosening the glute muscles, which can help with lower back pain. This stretch is also great for opening up the hips.

If you can't sit up to perform this movement, try a variation lying on the floor. Lie on your back and create the figure 4 with your legs as described above. Hold the supporting leg with both hands and bring both legs towards your body, you should feel a stretch in the glutes/hips of the non-supporting leg.

Single Leg Hamstring Stretch

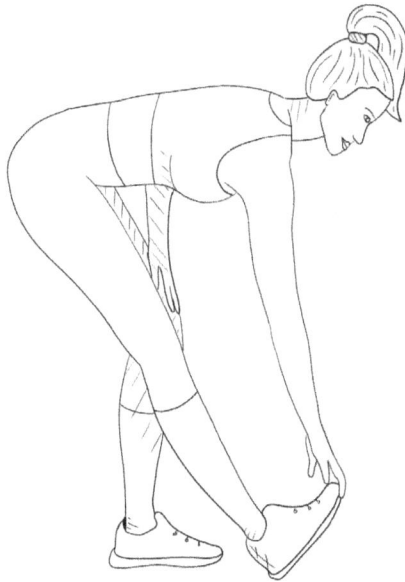

How to perform the Standing Single Leg Hamstring Stretch:

- **Step 1 – Get into position:** Stand tall with your back straight, abdominals engaged, shoulders down, and feet hip-width apart. Bring your right leg forward with your heel down, toes up, and leg straight.
- **Step 2 – Stretch:** Keep your back straight and your abs engaged. Bend your left knee as if you were sitting back and hinge your body forwards to feel the stretch. Keep supporting yourself with at least one hand on your thigh.

If you can't stand to perform this stretch, try it seated, as described below!

How to perform a Seated Single Leg Hamstring Stretch:

- **Step 1 – Get into position**: Sit on the edge of a sturdy chair and straighten your right leg in front of your body with your heel on the floor. Keep your left leg bent at a 90-degree angle.

- **Step 2 – Stretch:** Hold onto the chair with your left hand for support. Keep your back as straight as possible and bend forward, reaching down your right leg with your right hand. Stretch as far as is comfortable and then repeat with the other leg.

Primary Muscles Stretched: Your hamstrings! This stretch can also be a good stretch for your lower back.

Helps With: Increasing hamstring flexibility and improving the range of motion in your hips. Both of these benefits will help with daily tasks like bending down and walking.

After performing the stretches of choice, it's time to finish with a cooldown!

This cooldown sequence should be used after every strength training session. These movements can be performed sitting, standing, or lying down.

1. **Neck Rolls x 10 in each direction:** Let your chin slowly drop down to your chest. Circle your neck gently, taking the left ear to the left shoulder, then the head back, and then the right ear to the right shoulder. Repeat!

2. **Shoulder Rolls x 10 each direction:** Start by sitting up tall or lying down with an open chest, engaged core, and neutral spine. Pull your shoulders back and down and keep your gaze forward. To begin the shoulder roll, pull your shoulders up toward your ears as high as you can. Then squeeze your shoulder blades together to pull your shoulders back and down. Repeat 10 times, then another 10 times in the opposite direction.

3. **Handshakes x 30 seconds:** Begin by standing, sitting or lying down and hold your arms out on either side of your body. Shake your hands with relaxed wrists, letting any tension you feel run out through the bottom of your fingertips. Imagine any stress trickling out of the hands.

4. **Breathing Arm Raises x 5**: Take a deep breath and raise your arms from your sides to above your head. Exhale and let your arms float back down. Repeat 5 times.

Cool-down Visualization

It's easy to feel frustrated about your body not being able to move the way it used to when you were younger. But it's an incredible gift to be able to move at all, whether you're a 'senior' or not. Your cooldowns are a great time to develop gratitude for your body. Reflect on how well you've done by just making the choice to move your body, because it's something many people simply won't do.

Take a moment after your cool-down to breathe and cultivate that gratitude and pride for your body. When you inhale, praise yourself for the exercise you've just done, even just in your head. Even if it's just a small *'well done'* for getting up and moving. As you exhale, let go of any stress or tension you may be feeling. Tell yourself you will leave it with the workout that is now finished. Every next breath is a fresh one, bringing you energy and clean air, and anything toxic is getting pushed out as you exhale. Visualize the fresh air energizing you and giving you the boost you need for the rest of the day. Imagine any undesirable feelings leaving your body with your exhale. Tell your body that you are proud of it. Don't wait until you've reached your goal to be proud of yourself. Be proud of every step you take towards reaching that goal, no matter how small. Even if you don't feel it yet, **I** am proud of you. *Great work!*

Summary

You have just been given the tools you need to become a stronger, more energetic version of yourself. By doing some quick mobility work, a simple workout and cooldown sequence just a few times a week, you should be feeling less aches and pains and more fulfillment in no time.

Remember to use your workout time to focus on being thankful for all your body can do and feeling proud that you made the effort to work on yourself.

And remember;

"You are never too old to set another goal or to dream a new dream" - C.S Lewis.

Part 2. Chapter 8.

GLOSSARY OF STRENGTH TRAINING EXERCISES

Now that you have a great base from which to start your strength training journey and some practical ways to progress, you are well on your way to a happier and stronger you! So pack that catalog of walking sticks away; it won't be needed now!

Strength training is essential for building better body mechanics and can be done even if you've never trained in your life, so I do not doubt the incredible progress you're about to make. A study posted in *Aging Clinical and Experimental Research*[ix] concluded that doing at least one resistance or strength training session a week resulted in a 37% increase in muscle strength, a 7.5% increase in muscle mass, and a 58% increase in functional capacity which includes balance and mobility. With these motivating findings, I want to continue to help you reap the rewards of strength training.

If you are content with sticking to the previous chapter's training plan for the foreseeable that is absolutely fine, as you will make great progress and feel so much better within yourself, mind, body, and soul. But I wouldn't be satisfied if I didn't give those of you who want to progress further or crave more variety, some additional options.

In this next chapter, you will find a strength training exercise library bursting with movements you can try when you feel ready for a new challenge or want to try something different. Please only start trying these exercises and creating your own workouts once you have progressed your strength levels and feel comfortable with all of the movements in your provided exercise plan.

I would suggest sticking your exercise plan for the recommended 12 weeks at least before swapping out movements for ones in this glossary. Not only to avoid injury, but also to ensure progressive overload, which will be achieved through repeating the same movements using the progressions previously suggested.

Progressive overload is the best way to grow and get stronger, and simple is best when increasing your strength. I have to be honest and admit I have been guilty in the past of becoming bored with an exercise plan within a few weeks and have changed the exercises to keep it interesting. Unfortunately, in my haste for variety, I neglected progressive overload and failed to make good progress due to my impatience. Don't be like the younger me!

Trust the process and only add in different movements once you're already seeing results in terms of your strength and balance levels.

Start simple. I would recommend initially selecting a couple of movements from the glossary and adding them to your existing workout plan rather than switching to a combination of entirely new exercises - don't neglect the staples that improve and maintain your posture, strength and balance, etc.

If you do advance to the point of wanting to create your own workouts, here is a basic guide:

A good general structure for any workout is:

1. **Your mobility routine** (plus potentiation if you've reached a more advanced level).

2. **1 or 2 main compound movements**, aim for 8-12 repetitions of the same movement for 3 or 4 sets, with a 2-3 minute break in between sets. *When you can easily do 12 repetitions and no longer feel challenged, that's a good time to progress by adding small amounts of weight like dumbbells, a resistance band, or adding a more challenging progression of the movement. If adding weight you can lower the reps until you get more comfortable with the weight.*

3. **2 - 3 accessory movements.**

4. **A cool down and stretch.**

   After this glossary you will find some great workouts to help with certain ailments like back pain, poor core strength etc.. So please feel free to try those first if you're not yet confident enough to plan your own workout.

   If you do create any great workouts, please share them in our Facebook community 'Strength Training and Stretches for Over 60s', so that our members from all over the world can try your session!

This glossary contains:

Main Functional Compound Movements

A compound movement uses more than one muscle when performed. Compounds are functional movements and are my favorite to perform because of the full body workout they provide!

The movement pattern of many compound movements also mimics our daily movements which means improving our performance of the movement during the workout can help us to move better in our everyday lives!

Targeted Accessory Exercises

Targeted accessory exercises place the focus on different areas of the body. These are great to add into your routine as they can help to improve a specific area of weakness, which can help with muscular imbalances and overall functionality.

MAIN COMPOUND MOVEMENTS

Romanian Deadlifts

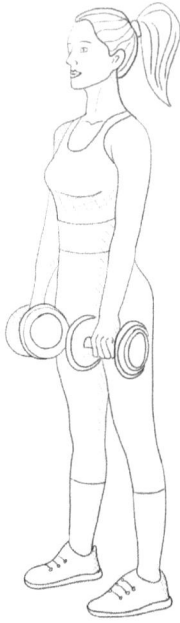

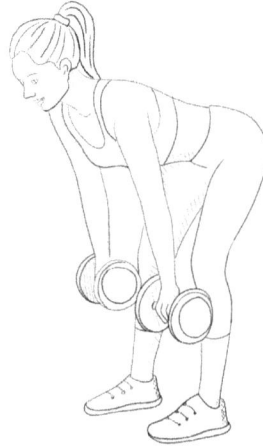

How to perform a Romanian Deadlift:
- **Step 1 – Get into position:** Stand with your feet shoulder-width apart and slightly bend your knees to prevent them from locking. Maintain this position the entire time. Your feet should be pointed forward, and you can hold some light dumbbells or household objects like bean cans to add some resistance. Pull your shoulder blades slightly back together to engage your upper back and ensure you're not hunching over.
- **Step 2 - Hinge forwards:** Keeping your knees slightly bent but not bending them any more, slowly hinge your body forward, whilst you push your hips backwards as far as you can and lower the objects in your hands down towards the floor, maintaining a straight and engaged back and straight arms - no hunching over! Try to keep the objects you're holding as close to the fronts of the legs as possible. Keep your head in line with your spine and stop when your upper body is parallel with the floor.

- **Step 3 – Pull upwards:** Keeping the muscles in your back, glutes and hamstrings engaged, use control and back/hamstring/glute strength to pull the upper body and any objects you're holding back up to the starting position. Maintain an engaged core when performing this exercise by taking a deep breath in between sets and imagine filling your tummy with air, hardening the outer layer. Engage your glutes as you stand up.

Primary Muscles Strengthened: Romanian deadlifts target mainly your glutes, hamstrings, and lower back muscles.

Helps With: Romanian deadlifts increase hip mobility, which is beneficial for any activities that require bending down and movements like sitting and standing up from a chair. They can also help with relieving lower back pain and stiffness by building a strong posterior chain and help to build great overall strength. They also help to strengthen the glutes, which are key muscles for walking, climbing and more, so there's no reason not to try this simple yet super effective compound movement!

Glute Bridge

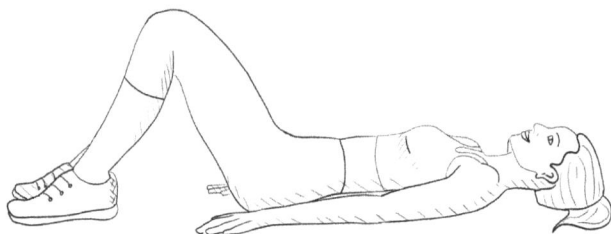

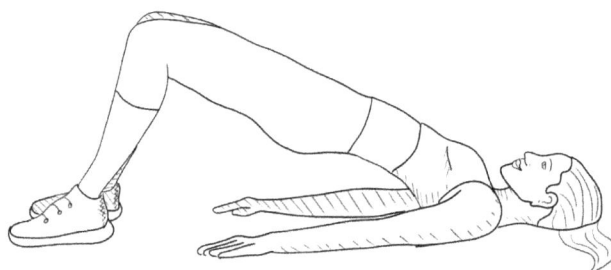

How to perform a Glute Bridge:
- **Step 1 – Lie on your back:** Lie flat on the floor with your arms by your sides and your legs extended. Bend your knees by placing your feet flat on the floor, about hip-width apart. Your spine should be in a neutral position and not arched. Keep your shoulders pulled back.
- **Step 2 – Engage your core:** Take a deep breath and brace your abdominal muscles, imagining filling your core up with air.
- **Step 3 – Lift your hips towards the ceiling:** Keeping your core engaged, drive your heels down into the floor and engage your glutes to raise your hips off the floor towards the ceiling. Your body should form a slanted line from your knees to your shoulders.
- **Step 4 – Hold:** Keep your shoulders rolled back and against the floor. Squeeze your glutes and keep a neutral back without arching. Hold this position for up to 5 seconds. The resistance should be felt in your hamstrings and glutes, not your lower back.

- **Step 5 – Lower your body:** Lower your body with control and rest for a few seconds before repeating.

Primary Muscles Strengthened:

The glutes are the main muscles worked in this movement, but the hamstrings and transverse abdominals (your deep core muscles that help with balance and stability) are also used.

Helps With:

Strengthening the gluteal muscles plays a role in increasing back and core stability which helps with posture and balance in everyday movements. Glutes are also a main muscle needed to walk forward, so strong glutes can contribute to walking with more ease.

Squat

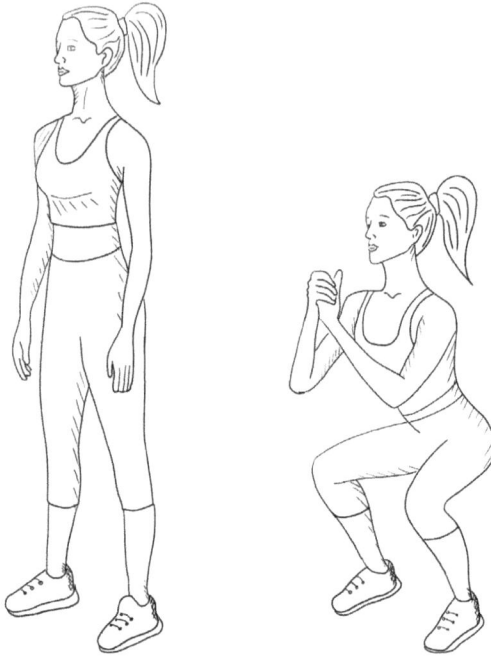

How to perform a Squat:

- **Step 1 – Get into position:** Start by standing tall with your feet hip-width apart. Your toes, knees and hips should all be facing forward.
- **Step 2 – Brace and squat:** Engage your core by taking a big deep breath and as you exhale, slowly begin to bend your knees and push your buttocks slightly backwards, as if you were going to sit down into a chair. Keep your weight evenly distributed between the front and back of your feet and only lower as far as is comfortable.
- **Step 3 – Stand:** Engage your glutes as you stand back up to complete the movement. Repeat.

Primary Muscles Strengthened:

Squats are a great compound movement that work almost every muscle in the body. The main muscles used are the glutes, hip flexors, and quads.

Helps With:

General overall strength. Squats are great for mirroring daily movements like sitting and standing up, making them a functional movement that also improves coordination. Squats should be a staple movement in your workout routine once you have sufficient core and general strength.

Try the 'Sit to Stand' on page 120 if you don't yet feel stable enough to try a squat!

Lunge

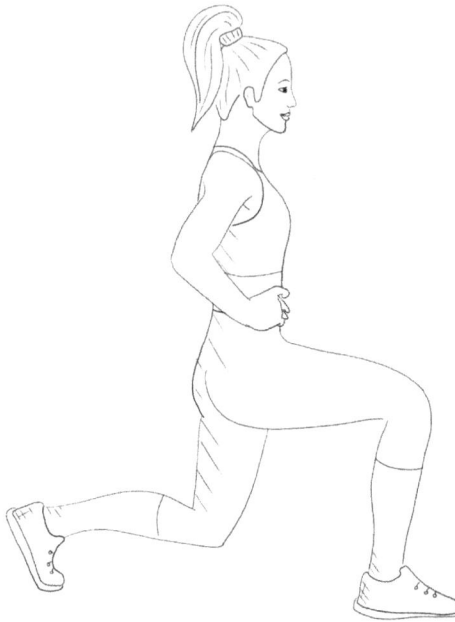

How to perform a Lunge:
- **Step 1 – Get into position:** Stand with your feet shoulder width apart and place your hands on your hips, or hold a small dumbbell (or small household object) in each hand if you'd like to add some resistance.
- **Step 2 – Lunge!:** Lunge one leg forwards and bend the knees to lower towards the floor. Tap the floor with your back knee and straighten your legs to finish the movement. Repeat!

Primary Muscles Worked: Lunges are a great all over body movement but they primarily target the legs, mainly the quads and hamstrings. The glutes are also targeted.

If you lean your torso further forward when performing a lunge you can target the glutes more. Or if you stay upright you can target the quads more. You can hold onto a chair whilst performing this movement if you require some support.

Helps With: Stronger legs will help with almost every daily movement - walking, standing and sitting and more. Lunges also strengthen the knee joints which will help with keeping you mobile and active. They are also great for core strength as your core muscles should kick in to help you balance, and better core strength = less risk of falling!

Push-ups

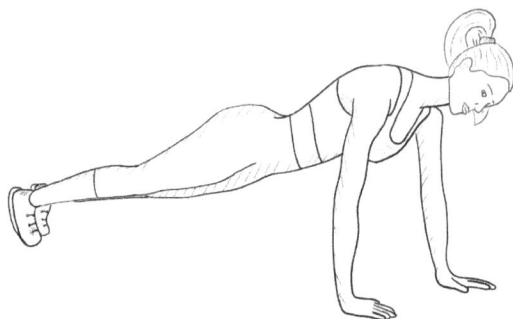

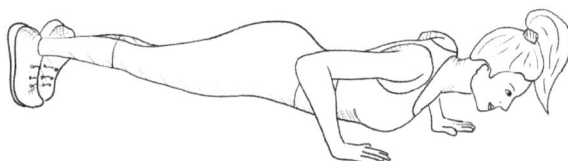

How to perform a Push-Up (advanced version):
- **Step 1 – Start on the ground:** Get onto the ground in a tabletop position, placing your hands slightly wider than shoulder-width apart and your knees on the floor hip width apart.
- **Step 2 – Plank position:** Move your legs backwards into a plank position. Keep your spine neutral, tucking your belly button in towards your spine, ensuring you don't arch your back.
- **Step 3 – Lower your body:** Bend your elbows to lower your body to the ground until your chest nearly touches the floor. Try to not let your body fall onto the floor as the resistance of keeping it off the ground is what will strengthen your muscles!
- **Step 4 – Push up:** Push yourself up by straightening your arms. Repeat!

How to perform a kneeling push-up (if a standard push up is too challenging):
- **Step 1 – Get down on the ground:** Get onto the ground in a tabletop position.

- **Step 2 – Get into position:** Lift your feet off the ground, keeping your knees on the floor as you shift your weight forwards onto your hands.
- **Step 3 – Lower your body:** Engage your core and glutes as you bend your elbows, lowering your body towards the ground until your chest nearly touches the floor. Keep your elbows at a 45-degree angle.
- **Step 4 – Push up:** Push yourself up again by straightening your arms. Repeat!

How to perform a wall push up (if a kneeling push up is too challenging):
- **Step 1 - Face a wall:** Stand with your feet shoulder width apart and place your hands on a wall in front of you with your arms straight.
- **Step 2 - Move towards the wall:** Engaging your core and bend your elbows as your body moves towards the wall, until your elbows are at a 45-degree angle.
- **Step 3 - Push up:** Push yourself away from the wall as you straighten your arms. Repeat!

Primary Muscles Strengthened:

Push-ups work the chest, shoulder muscles, triceps, and the abdominals.

Helps With:

Push-ups are great for building upper body strength, which can improve your posture and help with everyday tasks like lifting, reaching and carrying!

Good Mornings

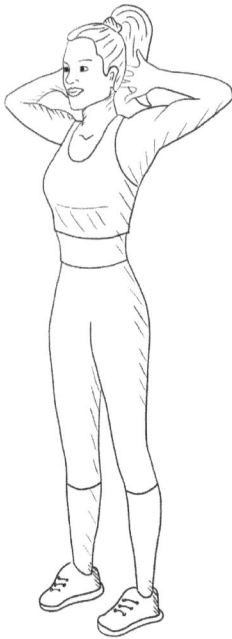

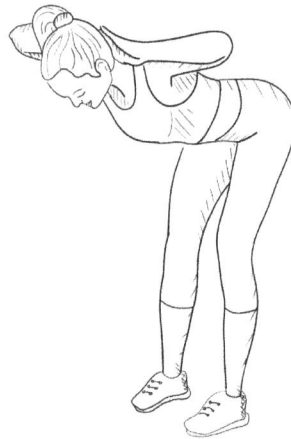

How to perform a Good Morning:
- **Step 1 – Get into position:** Place your hands on the back of your head and stand with your feet slightly wider than shoulder width apart with a small bend in your knees.
- **Step 2 – Hinge:** Engage your core and slowly hinge forward at the hips without bending your knees any more. Imagine your glutes being pushed backwards whilst keeping a straight back, no hunching! Keep bending over until your upper body is nearly parallel to the floor.
- **Step 3 – Pause and repeat:** Pause briefly in the hinged over position then raise your torso back up to the starting position to complete the movement.

Primary Muscles Strengthened:

The whole posterior chain, including your hamstrings, glutes, erector spinae, and lower back muscles.

Helps With: The hinge nature of good mornings helps to increase leg and back strength, which makes bending down and picking things up easier. Strong glutes and hamstrings will help with walking, climbing, sitting or standing so this is a great movement that will help you in your everyday life.

Wood Chops

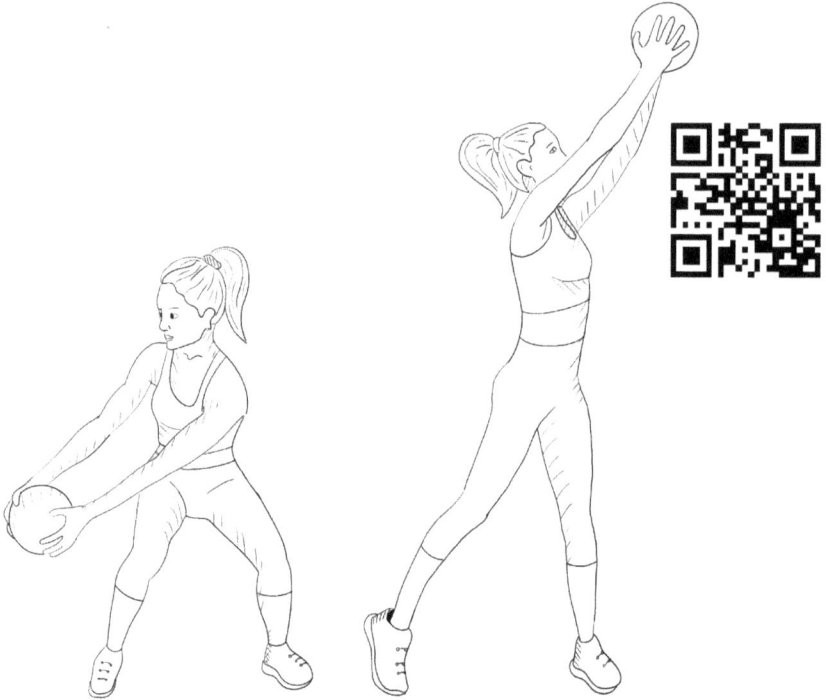

How to perform a Wood Chop:

- **Step 1 – Get into position:** Stand with your feet a little wider than shoulder-width apart and bend your knees slightly. Drive your feet into the ground for balance.
- **Step 2 – Hold a dumbbell, ball or other object:** Firmly hold your object with both hands - this should be light enough that you can lift and swing it without straining yourself but still adding some resistance.
- **Step 3 – Lift and twist:** Lift your arms and the object you're holding above your head to the left as you twist your hips and waist towards it. Shift your weight to your left foot with the heel of the right foot lifting off the floor as you lift the object.
- **Step 4 – Swing down with control:** Keeping your core engaged, pivot to the right, and swing the dumbbell diagonally down. The dumbbell should be level with your right knee. Turn your knees

and hips to the right as you bring the dumbbell down in one fluid motion whilst shifting your weight onto your right foot and peeling the heel of the left foot off the ground if needed.

- **Step 5 – Repeat:** Twist back up to the left with the object, being careful not to swing too fast, then swing back down to the right. Keep the motion slow and controlled and allow your core to feel the resistance. Once you've repeated the movement up to 10 times in one direction, try the same amount of reps on the other side!

If you can't stand, try performing a variation of this movement on a chair, by moving the object in your hands in the same way on each side for your desired number of reps. This will still provide a great core workout!

Primary Muscles Strengthened: This is a great movement for strengthening the core muscles. The thighs, calves and shoulder muscles are also involved as well as the hips for stabilizing. It's a great full body workout!

Helps With: Wood chops help to increase leg and core strength, making bending down, picking things up or any twisting movements easier. They're also great for improving coordination and balance.

Sit to Stand

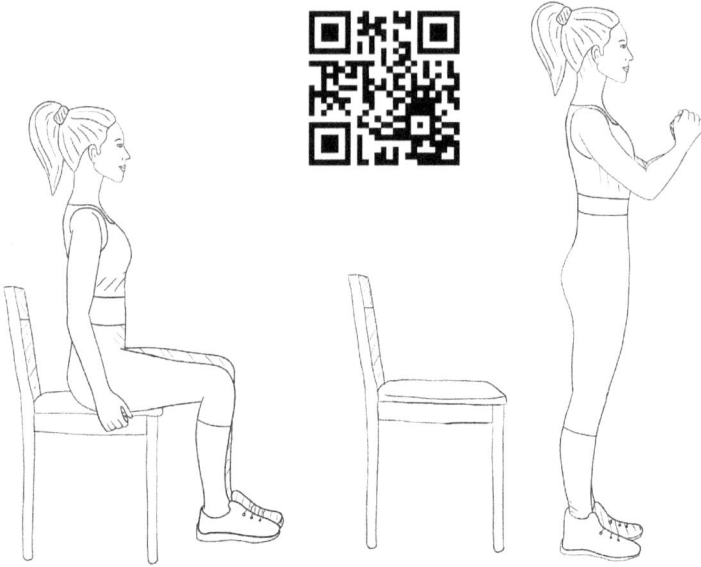

How to perform a Sit to Stand:

- **Step 1 - Sit:** Use a sturdy chair for this exercise. This movement can be performed supported (using your hands to push you up off the chair) or unsupported. Engage the trunk muscles by drawing the belly button towards the back and squeezing the glute muscles.
- **Step 2 - Stand:** With your feet placed apart, stand up in one motion.
- **Step 3 - Sit back down:** Slowly support yourself back to a seated position. Use your arms to guide you down to the seat until confident. Repeat!

Primary Muscles Strengthened:

Sit to stands are a great compound movement that works similar muscles to the squat. The main muscles used are the glutes, hip flexors, and quads.

Helps With:

Core strength, coordination and leg strength. The sit to stand is also a good alternative to a squat if you're not yet comfortable with the squat movement.

TARGETED ACCESSORY EXERCISES

Targeted Exercises for the Back

Your back muscles provide the structural support for your whole upper body. They contribute to a healthy posture and stabilize the spine. They also help you to bend forwards, turn sideways, and lift things off the ground.

In short, your back is very important, so let's strengthen it!

1. Lumbar Extensions

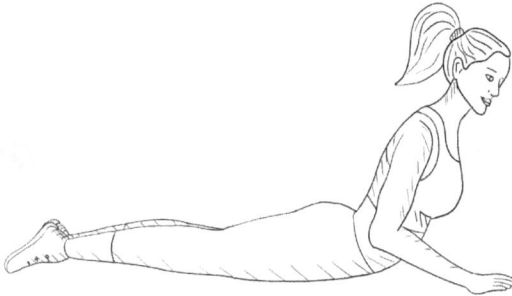

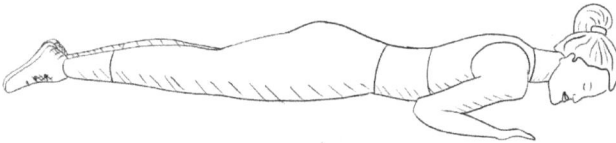

How to perform a Lumbar Extension:

- **Step 1 – Get into position:** Lie on your stomach on an exercise mat or soft floor. Place your forearms on the ground next to your head with your elbows bent. Gently pull your shoulders back together.

- **Step 2 –Extend:** Press your hands into the floor as you slowly lift your upper back off the floor, without overarching. Keep your neck and head neutral. Hold this position for 10-30 seconds as you take deep breaths. Lower to the starting position then repeat.

The first few times you try this movement, keep your forearms on the floor throughout. As you advance you can try improving your strength and flexibility even more by lifting the forearms off the floor and pushing your torso up further by pushing through your hands.

Primary Muscles Strengthened: The lower back muscles as well as the glutes. This movement also provides a nice stretch for the abdominal muscles.

2. Scapula Squeeze (can be performed standing, seated or lying down)

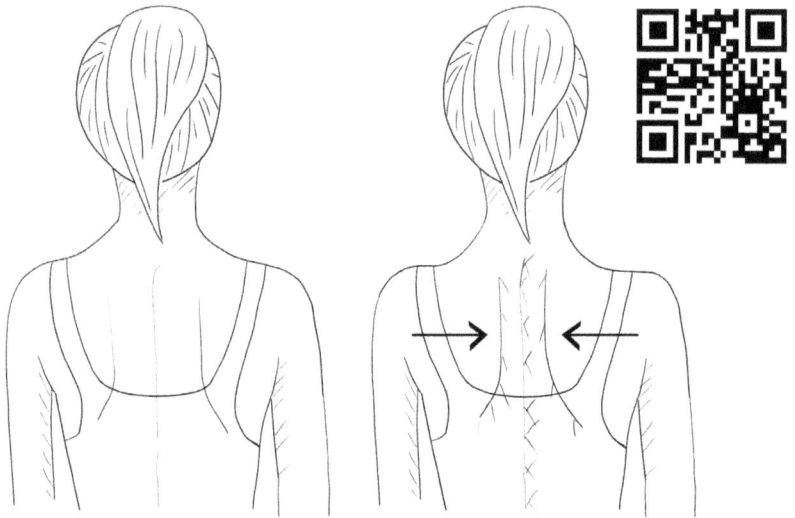

How to perform a Scapula Squeeze:
- **Step 1 – Stand, sit or lie down:** Stand with your feet hip-width apart, sit up straight on a chair with your feet flat on the floor, or lie down on a soft surface.
- **Step 2 – Squeeze:**

Option 1: Keep your arms down by your side and pull your shoulder blades back together. Hold for 10 seconds and return to the starting position.

Option 2: For a more advanced option that also gives the chest a small stretch, bend at your elbows and raise your arms to shoulder height with your palms facing forward. Moving your arms as far back as they'll go, squeeze your shoulder blades together. Hold for 10 seconds and return to the starting position.

Primary Muscles Strengthened: The central muscles of the back - the rhomboids. Which are very important for good posture!

3. Wall Angels

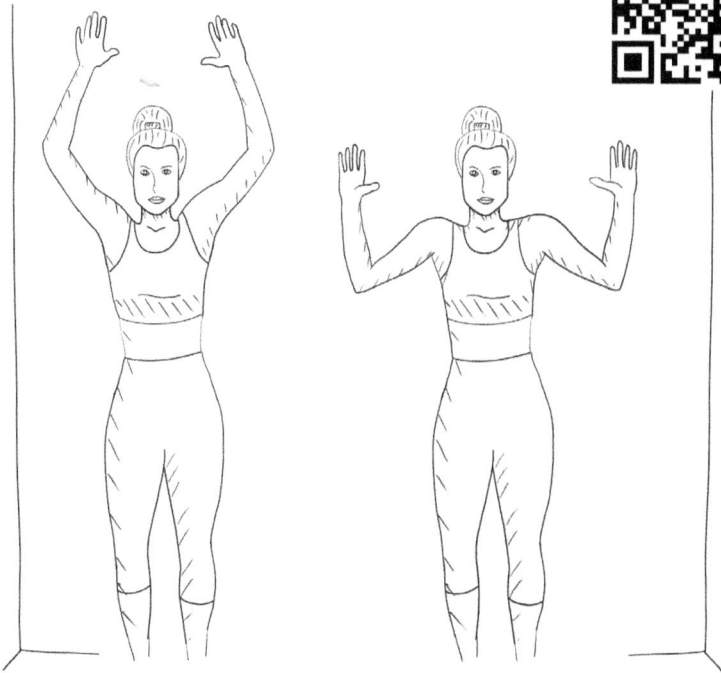

How to perform Wall Angels:

- **Step 1 – Get into position:** Stand with your head, shoulders, upper back, and buttocks pressed against the wall. Place the backs of your hands against the wall, and your forearms if you can, and slowly stretch your arms straight above your head to get into the starting position.

- **Step 2 – Carry out the move:** Squeeze your shoulder blades back and down together as you slide your arms downwards towards your shoulder line. Keep your body firmly pressed against the wall during this movement. When your elbows reach just below your shoulder line, pause for a few seconds then slide your arms back to the starting position.

If you can't stand up to perform this movement, perform the same movement pattern with your arms sat down or lying down!

Primary Muscles Strengthened: The postural muscles, chest muscles (pectoralis major and minor) and the large back muscle (latissimus dorsi). Strengthening these muscles can counteract a hunched over posture which can in time reduce back pain and help you stay upright!

Bent-Over Rows

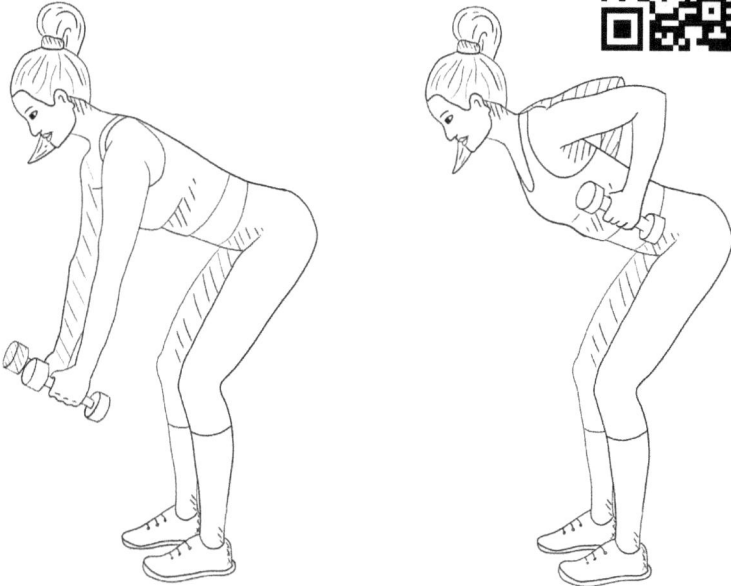

How to perform a Bent-Over Row:

- **Step 1 – Get into position:** Hold a dumbbell or small weighted household object in each hand and stand with your feet shoulder width apart. Slightly bend your knees and bend over whilst keeping your back straight. Your body should be almost parallel to the floor and your arms should be extended straight down with the dumbbells being aimed at the floor.

- **Step 2 – Row:** Bend your elbows to lift the dumbbells towards each side of your body whilst keeping your torso still. Squeeze your shoulder blades together and hold for a few seconds. Slowly lower the dumbbells back to the starting position. Repeat!

Perform this movement seated if you can't stand!

Primary Muscles Strengthened: The bent over row is a multi-jointed exercise that uses several different muscles. It improves strength mainly in the upper back and the latissimus dorsi ('the lats'), and also engages the hamstrings, arms and shoulders.

Helps With: Improving strength in the back, glutes, hamstrings, lats, and shoulders. A great movement that mimics bending over to lift everyday objects.

Targeted Exercises for the Core

A good level of core strength is vital for almost all of your everyday movements. From helping you sit or stand upright, to balancing, walking, lifting, bending and more. Your core is made up of your pelvic floor muscles, your abdominals, obliques, diaphragm, muscles that stabilize the spine, and more.

Though many compound movements are great for improving core strength, it's also beneficial to target certain areas of the core to improve its strength and stability, and now that you know just how many daily movements it effects, I hope you'll see it's not just beneficial to have a strong core, but vital if you want to stay strong and independent!

Here are some more exercises that target certain areas of the core!

(Though not repeated in this section, the dead bug (Page 74) and superman exercises (77) are amazing for your core, so you can refer back to those too!)

1. Ab Twists

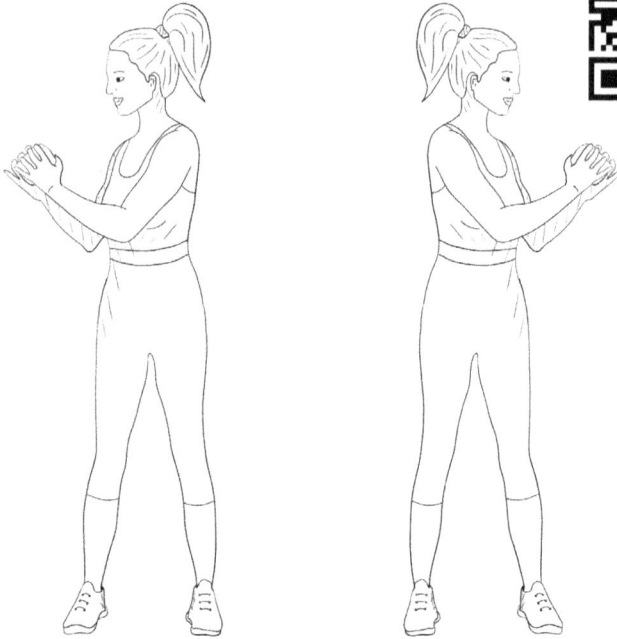

How to perform a Standing Ab Twist:
- **Step 1 – Get into position:** Stand with your legs hip-width apart. Make sure there is a soft bend in the knee. Hold a beach ball, medicine ball or other lightweight household object in your hands at chest level. Extend your arms outward holding your object.
- **Step 2 – Twist:** Keeping your pelvis stable, rotate your upper torso to the right, then back to the middle for a brief pause, then the left to complete one repetition, moving your arms and hands in the direction you're twisting. Be sure to keep your core engaged throughout the exercise and don't move too quickly so as to hurt your back.

If you can't stand, you can perform this same movement while sitting in a sturdy chair!

Primary Muscles Strengthened:

Side twists work mainly the rectus abdominis (the abs!), as well as the external and internal obliques. They're also great for getting some movement in the spine.

2. Seated Leans

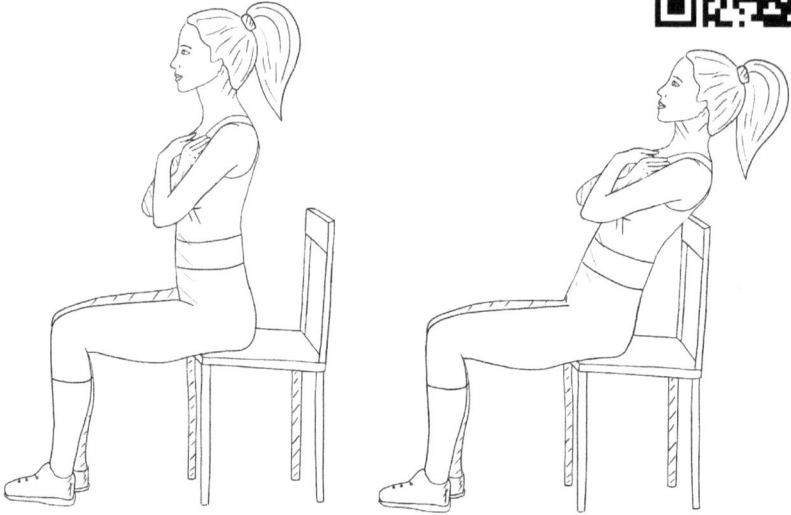

How to perform a Seated Lean:

- **Step 1 – Sit down:** Sit on the edge of a supportive chair in an upright position. Your shoulders should be pulled back and your pelvis slightly tucked under your body. Rest your hands gently on your thighs or for a more advanced version, crossed over on your shoulders.

- **Step 2 – Lean back:** Engage your core by contracting your abs and slowly lean back until your shoulder blades are gently touching the back of the chair. Do not put your full weight on the chair, allow your core to hold you in the position and keep your back as straight as possible. Allowing your core to feel this resistance is where you'll get the benefit of this movement. With your core still engaged, rise slowly back into an upright position.

Primary Muscles Strengthened: Seated leans work your main abdominal muscles as well as your lower back muscles.

3. Seated Ab Contraction

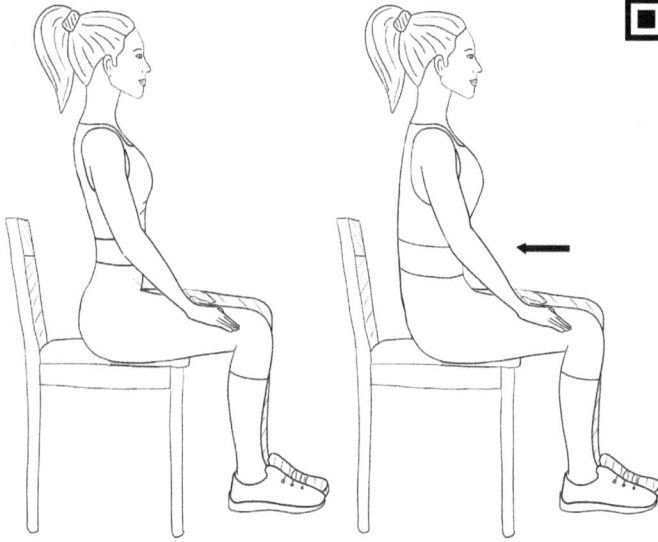

How to perform a Seated Ab Contraction:

- **Step 1 – Get into position:** Sit up straight on the edge of a chair with your feet planted firmly on the ground. Your shoulder blades should be pulled together with your hands resting on your knees.

- **Step 2 – Contract!:** Inhale as you brace and contract your abdominal and core muscles. Imagine that you're pulling your belly button toward your spine. Hold this for a few seconds and then release on an exhale (without slumping).

Primary Muscles Strengthened: The abdominal muscles!

4. Single Lying Leg Lifts

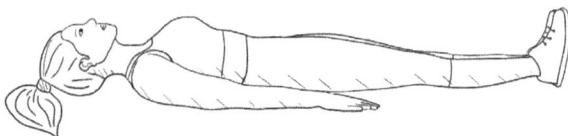

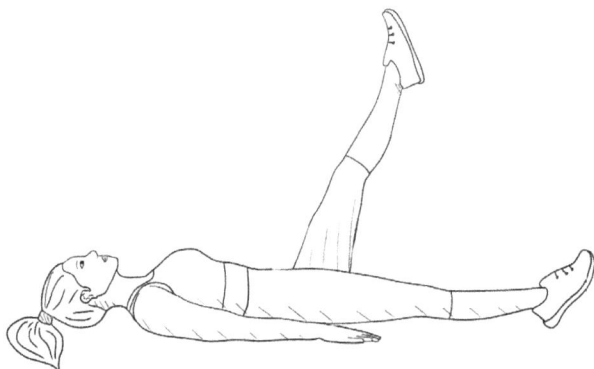

How to perform a Lying Leg Lift:
- **Step 1 – Get into position:** Lie down on your back with your arms next to your body and your legs straight. Alternatively, you can tuck your hands under your buttocks to relieve any pressure on your lower back.
- **Step 2 – Carry out the move:** Engage your abdominal muscles, keep your legs as straight as possible and lift one up to 90-degrees or as far as you can. Then slowly lower the leg back down until it's almost touching the floor. Hold for a moment and repeat. For a challenge, try this with both legs. If you find that lowering your legs all the way down is too uncomfortable on your lower back, you can lower them to around 45-degrees or whatever angle feels best for you!

Primary Muscles Strengthened:

The upper and lower abs. The hamstrings, quads, hip flexors, and lower back muscles are also targeted.

Targeted Exercises for the Hips and Glutes

Strong glutes and hips are essential for proper pelvic alignment, propulsion during running and walking, and standing and balancing. These muscles also support the lower back and help to prevent knee injuries.

As discussed earlier in this book, weak glutes or hips are also often the cause of lower back pain so it's really important to keep them strong!

1. Clam Shells

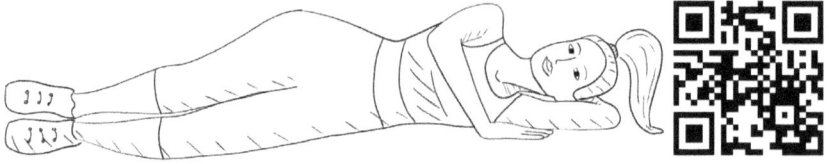

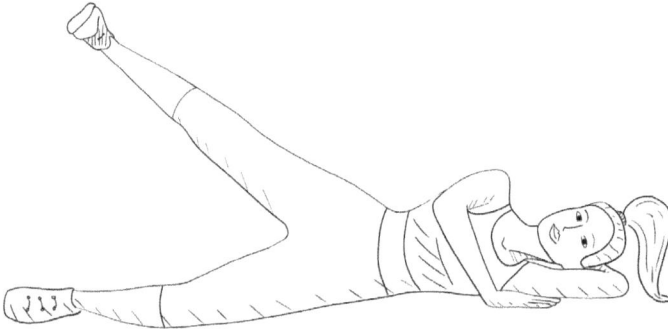

How to perform a Clam Shell:

- **Step 1 – Get into position:** Lie on your side with your legs on top of one another. Your knees should be slightly bent. Keep your feet together throughout the entire movement.

- **Step 2 – Carry out the movement:** Press your bottom leg firmly into the floor and, with your heels pressed together, squeeze your glute muscles to raise your top knee toward the ceiling, imagining a clam shell opening up! Raise the knee as high as possible without letting your pelvis rock backward or forwards. Pause for a second, then lower your leg down again. Repeat for your chosen amount of repetitions then repeat on the other leg!

Primary Muscles Strengthened:

Clam shells work mainly the gluteus medius, the muscle on the outer edge of your buttocks. These muscles are responsible for stabilizing the pelvis and are a key muscle involved in any side-wards movement. The gluteus maximus is also targeted. Stronger glutes can reduce back and knee pain by taking some of the load when performing many daily movements.

2. Glute Kicks-Backs/Donkey Kicks

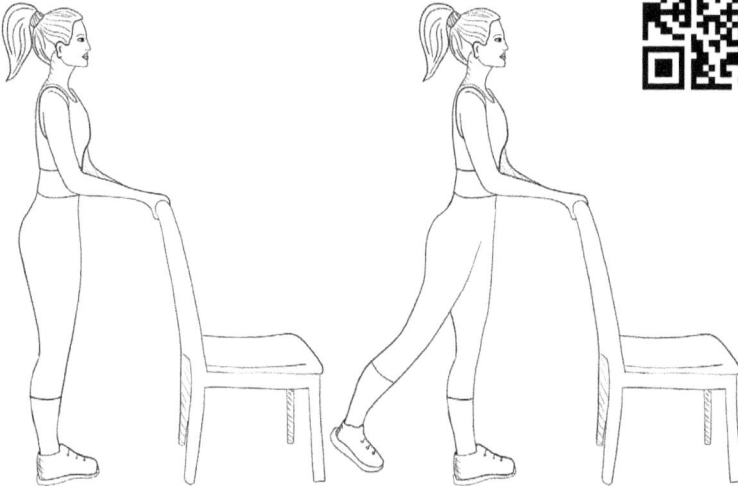

How to perform a standing Glute Kick-Back/Donkey Kick:
- **Step 1 – Get into position:** Stand with your feet shoulder width apart and hold onto a strong surface. Your spine should be straight and your core muscles engaged.
- **Step 2 – Gently kick backwards:** Extend one leg backwards behind your body as you feel the glute on your working leg engage. Hold this position for a few deep breaths as you feel the resistance on your glute, then return the leg to the starting position. Repeat for your chosen amount of repetitions then try on the other leg!

How to perform a floor Glute Kick-Back/Donkey Kick:

If you can't stand up, you can try a variation of this movement in a table top position!
- **Step 1 – Get into position:** Get into a tabletop position with your knees and hands on the floor. Imagine pulling your belly

button into your spine to engage your core, without arching the back.

- **Step 2 – Gently kick upwards :** Lift your left leg up and back until your thigh is parallel with the floor. The sole of your foot should be facing the ceiling. Contract your glute at the top and hold the position for a second or two. Return to the starting position without the knee touching the floor and repeat. Once you have completed a set with one leg, swap and repeat on the other leg!

Primary Muscles Strengthened: Glute kick-backs or "donkey kicks" are a great exercise for working all parts of your glutes, including the gluteus maximus, gluteus medius, and gluteus minimus. The kick-back also works your hamstrings and is great for improving balance and coordination.

3. Lateral Leg Raises

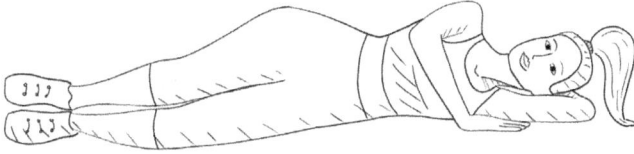

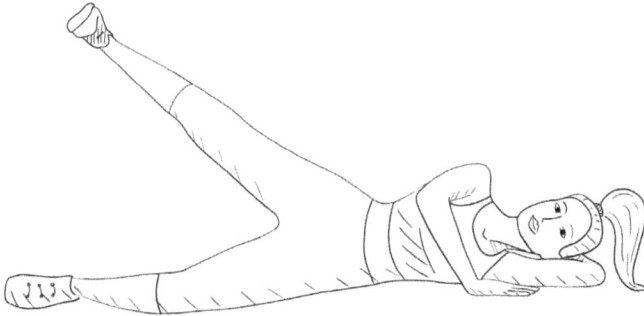

How to perform a Lateral Leg Raise:

- **Step 1 – Get into position:** Lie on your side on a soft surface. Prop yourself up on your elbow and place your hand under your head for support. Keep your spine neutral and tuck your chin in slightly towards your chest. Place your other hand in front of your waist or chest on the floor to stabilize you. Your legs should be fully extended and stacked on top of each other. Your body should form a straight line.

- **Step 2 – Raise!:** Engage your core and lift your top leg up as far as you can. Pause at the top of the movement then slowly lower your leg down again. Repeat for your chosen number of repetitions then turn over and repeat on the other side.

Primary Muscles Strengthened:

Lateral leg raises activate various muscle groups throughout the body, including the core, glutes, hip flexors, hamstrings, and lower back muscles.

Targeted Exercises for the Legs

Strong leg muscles make daily activities much easier. They help with balance and mobility, not to mention walking, climbing, bending and so many other important movements.

Targeted leg exercises ensure you're strengthening the individual leg muscles which will contribute to overall leg strength.

1. Leg Extensions

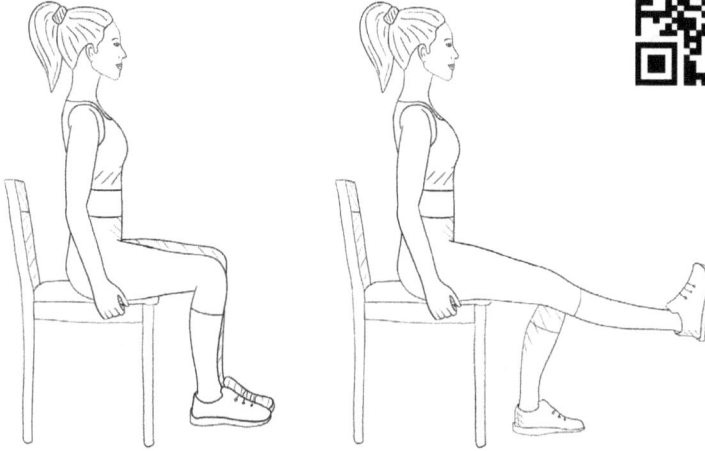

How to perform a Leg Extension:

- **Step 1 – Sit down:** Sit up straight in a chair with your upper body against the back of the chair. Ensure your shoulders are pulled back and look forward with your head in a neutral position. You can place your hands by your sides for stability. Your knees should be hip-width apart and at a 90-degree angle.

- **Step 2 – Extend!:** Keeping your core engaged, inhale and then exhale as you straighten one knee, extending your leg out to the front of you in a slow and steady motion. Your leg should finish parallel with the floor. Once your leg is extended, hold for at least two seconds to allow your quads to engage before slowly lowering it to the starting position. Repeat on the other leg!

Primary Muscles Strengthened: The quadriceps!

2. Calf Raises

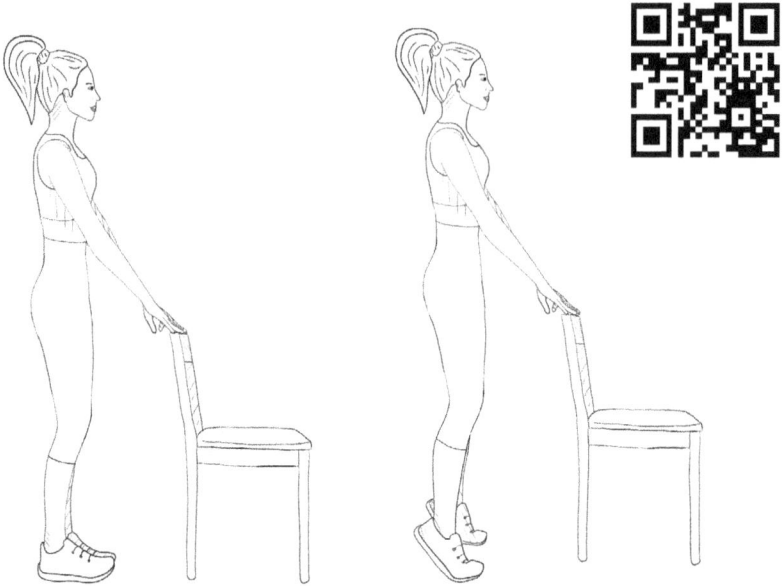

How to perform a standing supported Calf Raise:
- **Step 1 – Find a stable surface:** Find a sturdy platform and place your hands on it, standing with your feet shoulder width apart.
- **Step 2 – Raise:** Slowly rise up onto your toes and push your heels up as far as you can go. Then lower your heels back down and repeat.

A more advanced version of the calf raise is to place your toes on a step whilst holding onto a wall next to it for stability, and perform the calf raise with the added depth.

*If you can't stand you can also perform seated calf raises as shown in the video linked to this QR code:  *

Primary Muscles Strengthened: The clue is in the name! Calf raises work your calf muscles, which actually comprise three muscles - your gastrocnemius, soleus and plantaris!

3. Seated Leg Curls

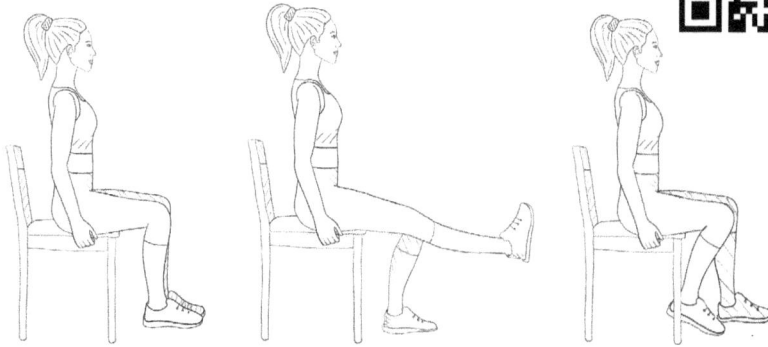

How to perform a Leg Curl:

- **Step 1 - Sit down and extend:** Sit on the edge of a bed or chair with one foot placed on the ground for support and one leg extended with the knee straight (like you're performing a leg extension).

- **Step 2 - Curl:** Whilst bending the knee on the extended leg, pull the heel under the chair or bed frame by contracting the muscle on the back of the thigh. Hold for 5 seconds before relaxing slowly and under control. Repeat on the other leg and perform up to 12 alternate leg curls. Skip this movement if you can't sit up!

Primary Muscles Strengthened: The hamstrings!

Targeted Exercises for the Arms

Having strong arms can allow you to maintain good general strength when it comes to lifting everyday objects. By regularly performing arm strengthening movements you're also keeping your elbows and shoulders mobile!

1. Bicep Curls

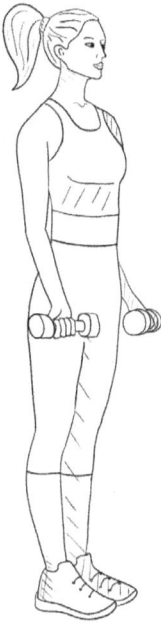

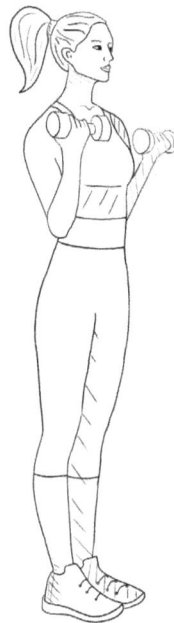

How to perform a Bicep Curl:

- **Step 1 – Get into position:** Start by standing, sitting or lying down with a dumbbell or other small household objects (like a bean can) in each hand. Your feet should be shoulder-width apart, with your arms down by your side and your forearms extended slightly in front of the body.

- **Step 2 – Curl!:** Bring the dumbbells in to touch the top of your arms in a controlled motion by bending your elbows. Once you reach the top, reverse the curl and slowly lower down to the starting position allowing yourself to feel the resistance in your biceps. Repeat!

Primary Muscles Strengthened:

The Biceps!

2. Tricep Kickbacks

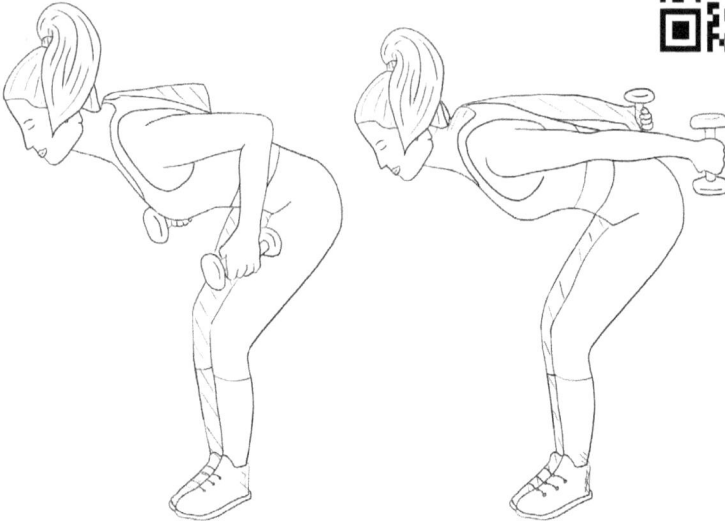

How to perform a Tricep Kickback:

- **Step 1 – Get into position:** Stand or sit with your feet shoulder-width apart and keep your back straight as you bend forward. Hold a dumbbell or bean can in each hand and bend your elbows as you pull your upper arms in line with your body, pulling your shoulder blades slightly back together.
- **Step 2 – Kickback!:** Engage your tricep muscles as you straighten your arms backwards, keeping your upper arms in the same position. Hold for 2 seconds before bending your elbows to bring your arms back to the starting position.

Primary Muscles Strengthened: The Triceps - located in the back of the upper arm.

Targeted Exercises for the Shoulders

Strong shoulder muscles contribute to good posture and help with lifting and carrying. Shoulder injuries due to inactivity are very common, so it's important to keep the shoulder joints moving and the muscles strong!

1. Lateral Raises

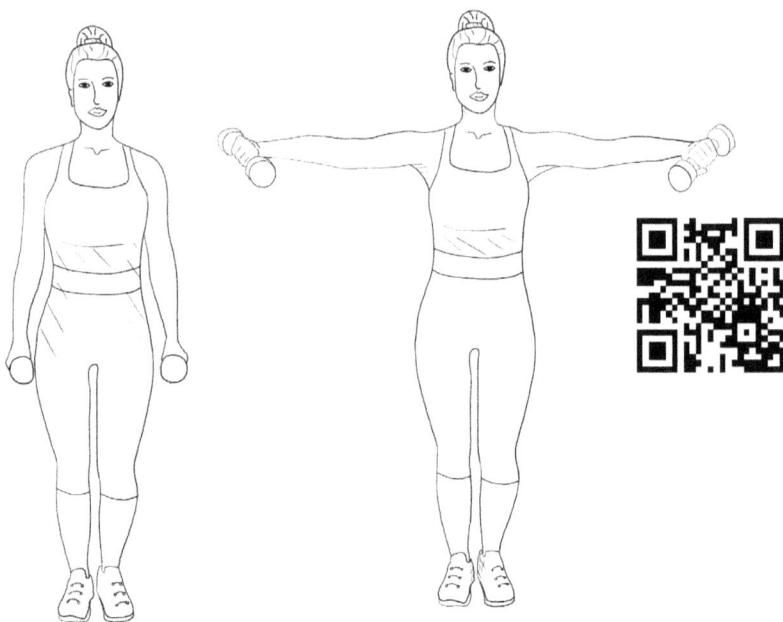

How to perform a Lateral Raise:

- **Step 1 – Get into position:** If you are using weights, choose dumbbells/light objects that you can easily move around without straining. Stand tall with your feet shoulder-width apart and a dumbbell (or not) in each hand. Your arms should be hanging by your sides. Pull your shoulders back and engage your core.
- **Step 2 – Raise!:** Raise your arms simultaneously out to the side, with a slight bend in the elbows. Start by only raising by a few inches if you can't bring the arms very far up yet. Pause for a few seconds. Lower the weights down slowly and return to the starting position.

Primary Muscles Strengthened: Your shoulder muscles as well as your latissimus dorsi and upper trapezius.

2. Military Press

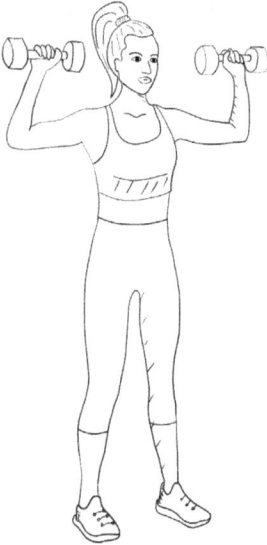

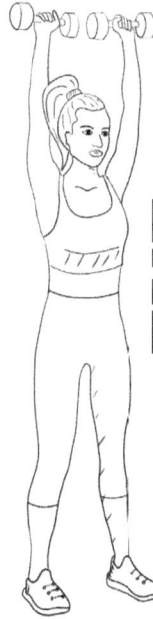

How to perform a Military Press:

- **Step 1 – Get into position:** Stand with your feet shoulder width apart or sit on a solid chair with your lower back firmly pressed against the back of the chair. Hold dumbbells (or other household objects like bean cans) in your hands with your elbows bent and your upper arms in line with your shoulders.

- **Step 2 – Press:** Lift the dumbbells up above your head in a controlled manner until your arms extend fully, making sure you do not lock out your elbows. Hold the weight overhead for a second, then lower the dumbbells back to the starting height. Repeat!

Primary Muscles Strengthened: A military press, also known as a shoulder press or overhead press, focuses mainly on the deltoids and other shoulder muscles, as well as the triceps and the trapezius muscles. The movement uses the same muscles that you'd use if you were lifting things above your head to put in high cupboards, so strengthening these muscles will come in handy in your day-to-day life!

Targeted Exercises for the Chest

Strong chest muscles help to stabilize the shoulder joints and play a big part in improving your posture. Lengthening and strengthening the chest muscles also helps to support deeper breathing.

Your chest also helps with pushing movements so it's important to keep it strong so that you can continue performing many daily movements with ease!

1. Plate Pinch Press (Svend Press)

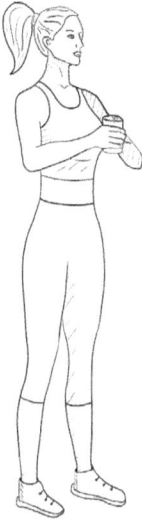

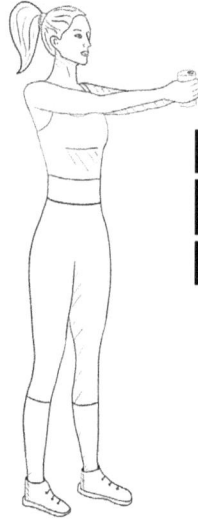

How to perform a Svend Press:

- **Step 1 – Get into position:** Hold a dumbell, medicine ball or other small/thin lightly weighted object with both hands. Stand strong with your feet shoulder-width apart. Bring the object you're holding to the middle of your chest with your fingertips pointing away from your body. Press your palms together as hard as you can against the object. Ensure that your shoulder blades are pulled back and down and that you're not hunched over. Your chest must be up and open so that you are properly isolating your chest muscles.

- **Step 2 – Press:** Use a controlled motion to extend your arms forward away from your chest, whilst pressing your hands towards each other onto the object as firmly as possible. Once your arms are fully extended, begin bringing the object back to the starting position. Repeat!

Primary Muscles Strengthened:

The plate pinch press exercise works the upper and lower pectoral muscles.

2. Chest Press

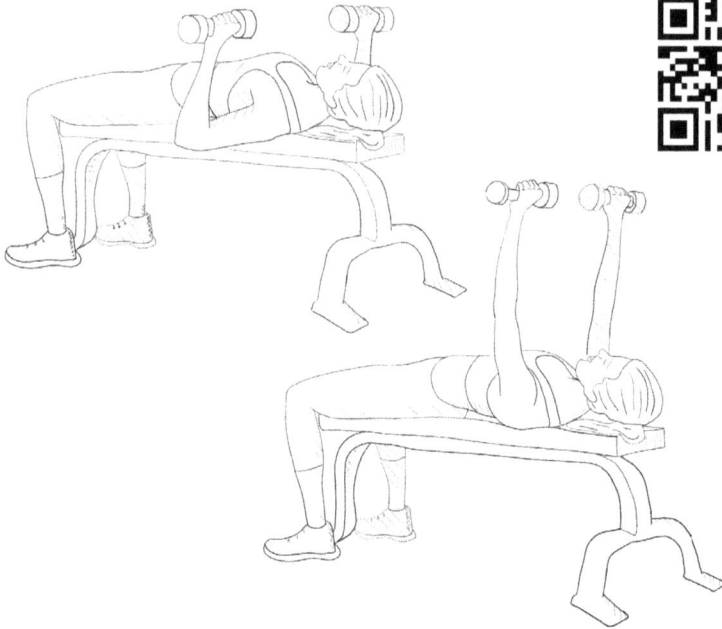

How to perform a Chest Press:

- **Step 1 – Get into position:** Lie flat on your back on a bench (or if at home with no bench, on the floor) with your knees bent and feet on the floor.

- **Step 2 – Brace your body:** Tuck your shoulder blades behind your back, this will help keep your arms from flaring out too much. Press down into the floor with your feet while you create a small arch in your back - don't hyperextend! Your bodyweight should be resting on your buttocks and the back of your shoulders.

- **Step 3 – Raise your dumbbells:** Holding a dumbbell or other household object (like a bean can) tight in each hand, raise your hands above your head with your hands slightly wider than shoulder-width apart.

- **Step 4 – Lower the weight:** Lower the dumbbells to just above chest level in a controlled motion (or as far down as the floor allows if doing these without a bench). Maintain good pressure through your feet the entire time.

- **Step 5 – Press the weight back up:** Then press the weight back up in an explosive action. Exhale at the end of every repetition and repeat!

Primary Muscles Strengthened: The pectorals (chest muscles), the shoulders, and the triceps.

Now what?

As mentioned at the start of this chapter, these strength training exercises can be used to add variety to your workout plan to keep things fun and help you to progress in different ways. Or you could mix them together based on physical weaknesses you currently have so that you can target the areas in your body that need strengthening the most!

On the following pages are some examples of tailored workouts to help with specific areas of weakness. You can use these as they are, or use them as a general guideline/inspiration for creating your own workouts. Remember that progressive overload is key for strength building, so with any workout plan you partake in you should aim for at least 2-3 sessions each week with some of the same exercises and small challenges added along the way.

Please make sure you add a warm up/mobility sequence before each workout and a cooldown after!

TAILORED WORKOUTS

Please note, these workouts should only be attempted once you have built up a good amount of general strength, at least after 12 weeks of your provided exercise plan!

Strong Back Workouts:

A strong back will have you standing strong and upright for the years to come. Back pain is extremely common but it doesn't need to be! Take care of your back so that you can stay mobile and active forever!

Workout 1)

- Lying Knee to Chest - 10 each leg x 3 (1-2 minute rest inbetween sets)
- Glute Bridges - 3x10 (2-3 minute rest inbetween sets)
- Cat/Cow Stretches - 3x10 (1-2 minute rest inbetween sets)
- Lumbar Extensions - 3x3 (holding the extension for 10 secs each time) (1-2 minute rest inbetween sets)
- Scapula Squeeze - Hold for 10 secs each time x 5

Workout 2)

- Cat/Cow Stretches - 3x10 (1-2 minute rest inbetween sets)
- Romanian Deadlifts - 3x10 - adding a small weight with dumbbells or bean cans if comfortable (2-3 minute rest inbetween sets)
- Glute Kick-Backs - 3x10 (2-3 minute rest inbetween sets)

- Wall Angels - 3x10 (1-2 minute rest inbetween sets)
- Lumbar Extensions - 3x3 with a 10 second pause when extended (1-2 minute rest inbetween sets)

Workout 3)

- Cat/Cow Stretches - 3x10 (1-2 minute rest inbetween sets)
- Romanian Deadlifts- 3x10 - adding a small weight with dumbbells or bean cans if comfortable (2-3 minute rest inbetween sets)
- Glute Bridges - 4x10 (2-3 minute rest inbetween sets)
- Lying Clam Shells - 3x10 each side (1-2 minute rest inbetween sets)

Workout 4)

- Lumbar Extensions - 3x3 with a 10 second pause when extended (1-2 minute rest inbetween sets)
- Good Mornings - 3x10 (2-3 minute rest inbetween sets)
- Glute Kickbacks - 3x10 each side (2-3 minute rest inbetween sets)
- Cat/Cow Stretches - 3x10 (1-2 minute rest inbetween sets)
- Figure 4 Glute Stretch - 3x10 seconds each leg (1-2 minute rest inbetween sets)

Workout 5)

- Superman progression of your choice - 3x10 each side (1-2 minute rest inbetween sets)
- Good Mornings 3x10 (2-3 minute rest inbetween sets)
- Wall Angels - 3x10 (1-2 minute rest inbetween sets)
- Bent Over Rows - 3x10 (1-2 minute rest inbetween sets)
- Clam Shells - 3x10 each side (1-2 minute rest inbetween sets)

Stronger Core Workouts:

A strong core is needed for everything from holding your body upright, to allowing you to twist, turn, lift and more!

Balance is achieved by our muscles being strong enough to hold us up, so having a strong core will also greatly reduce the risk of falls.

Workout 1)

- 4 Point Shoulder Taps - 3x10 each side (1-2 minute rest inbetween sets)
- Squats or Sit to Stands - 3x10 (2-3 minute rest inbetween sets)
- Seated Slow Lean Backs - 3x8 (1-2 minute rest inbetween sets)
- Lying Leg Raises - 3x10 each leg (1-2 minute rest inbetween sets)
- Superman progression of your choice - 3x10 each side (1-2 minute rest inbetween sets)

Workout 2)

- Wood Chops - 3x10 each side (1-2 minute rest inbetween sets)
- Ab Twists - 4x10 (1-2 minute rest inbetween sets)
- Push Ups - 3x10 (pick the difficulty level most suitable) (2-3 minute rest inbetween sets)
- Lying Leg Raises - 3x10 each leg (1-2 minute rest inbetween sets)
- Superman progression of choice - 3x10 each side (1-2 minute rest inbetween sets)

Workout 3)

- Shopping Bag Hold - 3x10 each side (1-2 minute rest inbetween sets)
- Wood Chops - 3x10 each side (1-2 minute rest inbetween sets)
- Superman progression of choice - 3x10 each side (1-2 minute rest inbetween sets)
- Seated Slow Lean Backs - 3x8 (1-2 minute rest inbetween sets)
- Single Knee Lift and Tap - 3x10 each leg (1-2 minute rest inbetween sets)

Workout 4)

- 1 Leg Balance - 3x8-10 each leg (1-2 minute rest inbetween sets)

- Shopping Bag Carry - 3x10 steps each side (1-2 minute rest inbetween sets)
- Squats or Sit to Stands - 3x10 (2-3 minute rest inbetween sets)
- Lying Leg Raises - 3x10 each leg (1-2 minute rest inbetween sets)
- Dead Bug progression of your choice - 3x10 each side (1-2 minute rest inbetween sets)

Workout 5)

- Wood Chops - 3x10 each side (1-2 minute rest inbetween sets)
- Sit to Stand - 3x10 (2-3 minute rest inbetween sets)
- 1 Leg Balance - 3x8-10 each leg (1-2 minute rest inbetween sets)
- Push Ups - 3x10 (pick the difficulty level most suitable) (2-3 minute rest inbetween sets)
- Lying Leg Raises - 3x10 each leg (1-2 minute rest inbetween sets)

Stronger Legs Workouts

The following workouts are great for preventing knee pain and helping with everyday movements like climbing stairs and walking. We need our legs to keep doing most of the things we love, so take care of them now so that you can continue being active later!

Workout 1)

- Standing Knee Lift and Tap - 2 minutes alternating sides
- Sit to Stands - 2x10 (1-2 minute rest inbetween sets)
- Squats 4x10 (2-3 minute rest inbetween sets) (if you can't yet perform squats, perform two more sets of 10 sit to stands instead).
- Seated Leg Extensions 3x10 (1-2 minute rest inbetween sets)
- Supported Calf Raises 3x10 (1-2 minute rest inbetween sets)

Workout 2)

- Standing Knee Lift and Tap - 2 minutes alternating sides
- Wood Chops - 3x10 each side (1-2 minute rest inbetween sets)

- Squats 4x10 (2-3 minute rest inbetween sets) (if you can't yet perform squats, perform two more sets of 10 sit to stands instead).
- Lunges 3x8 each leg (1-2 minute rest inbetween sets)
- Seated Leg Curls 3x10 (1-2 minute rest inbetween sets)
- Seated Leg Extensions 3x10 (1-2 minute rest inbetween sets)

Workout 3)

- Standing Knee Lift and Tap - 2 minutes alternating sides
- Wood Chops - 3x10 each side (1-2 minute rest inbetween sets)
- Romanian Deadlifts 4x10 (2-3 minute rest inbetween sets)
- Lunges - 4x1o each leg (1-2 minute rest inbetween sets)
- Seated Leg Extensions - 3x10 (1-2 minute rest inbetween sets)

Workout 4)

- 1 Leg Balance - 3x10 each leg (1-2 minute rest inbetween sets)
- Sit to Stand - 3x10 (1-2 minute rest inbetween sets)
- Supported Calf Raises - 3x10 (1-2 minute rest inbetween sets)
- Seated Leg Extensions - 3x10 (1-2 minute rest inbetween sets)
- Lying Lateral Leg Raises - 3x10 (1-2 minute rest inbetween sets)

Workout 5)

- Shopping Bag Carry - 3x10 each side (1-2 minute rest inbetween sets)
- 1 Leg Balance - 3x10 each leg (1-2 minute rest inbetween sets)
- Lunges - 4x10 each leg (2-3 minute rest inbetween sets)
- Standing Glute Kick-Back - 3x10 (1-2 minute rest inbetween sets)
- Supported Calf Raises - 3x10 (1-2 minute rest inbetween sets)

Sciatica Workout

'Sciatica' is a pain that is felt along the path of the sciatic nerve. It is common not just in the aging population but in people of all ages, especially pregnant women. The sciatic nerve runs from your lower back to your feet and is irritated when compressed or rubbed on, which can happen due to a variety of reasons. It is always advised to seek a medical professional's help to get a treatment plan to help with sciatica, but as I've seen people very close to me suffer with this, I couldn't not include some pain relieving exercises in this book. So alongside a treatment plan from your doctor, here are some routines to try if you suffer with sciatica pain!

Sciatica Workout 1)

- Windshield Wipers - starting with just gentle knee rocks side to side first until comfortable 4x10 (1-2 minute rest inbetween sets)
- Glute Bridge - 4x10 (2-3 minute rest inbetween sets)
- Figure 4 Glute Stretch - 3x10-30 seconds each side (1-2 minute rest inbetween sets)
- Knee to Chest Stretch (bringing your opposite knee towards your opposite shoulder instead of directly up onto the body) - 3x30 seconds each leg, alternating legs.

Sciatica Workout 2)

- Glute Bridge 4x10 (2-3 minute rest inbetween sets)
- Knee to Chest Stretch (but bring your opposite knee towards your opposite shoulder instead of directly up onto the body) - 3x30 seconds each leg, alternating legs.
- Standing Hamstring Stretch 3x10 secs each leg, alternating legs
- Figure 4 Glute Stretch 3x15-30 seconds each side
- Childs Pose 4x30 seconds

Pelvic Floor Workout

Our pelvic floor muscles can weaken with age, largely due to repeated bad pelvic floor habits, like not activating the muscles enough with exercises, or holding our pee in too long! Though small leaks are nothing to be ashamed of, they can understandably cause a lot of embarrassment and distress for older adults (or anyone, for that matter!). If you're wanting to remain dignified and independent, a strong pelvic floor is key! Below is a short pelvic floor workout that when repeated regularly, can tighten the pelvic floor muscles.

It would be beneficial to perform Kegels (described below) everyday alongside your workout routine even if you decide against the full pelvic floor workout.

Pelvic Floor Workout:

Kegels:

Squeeze your pelvic floor muscles 10-15 times. Imagine trying to hold in a pee if you struggle to know how to squeeze the muscles!

Once you are able to perform the contraction, try adding a few second pause each time you contract. Once you work up to 15 repetitions (or how many you're able to perform), take a rest break for 1 minute before repeating.

Then perform:

Glute Bridges 4x10 (2-3 minute rest inbetween sets)

Seated Ab Contractions - 4x10 (1-2 minute rest inbetween sets)

Lying Leg Raises - 3x10 each leg (1-2 minute rest inbetween sets)

Better Balance Workouts

Lack of balance is something that many older adults struggle with and it can cause what is a lot of seniors' biggest fear: falling. But poor balance doesn't necessarily have to come with age, it is caused more by inactivity, and the muscle imbalances and lack of coordination and strength that comes with that. Building up a good base level of core strength from the exercise plan in Part 2. Chapter 6, will help you to improve your balance so please allow that to work its magic before trying something new!

But when you're ready for a new challenge or some variety, here are some different workouts to try that really focus on strengthening your muscles and your core, improving your balance and reducing your risk of falling.

Balance Workout 1

- Shopping Bag Carry - 10 steps each direction x 4 (1-2 minute rest inbetween sets)
- Supported 1 Leg Balance - 3x10 seconds each leg (1-2 minute rest inbetween sets)
- Sit to Stand - 4x10 (2-3 minute rest inbetween sets)
- Standing Lateral Leg Raise 3x8-10 each leg (1-2 minute rest inbetween sets)
- Ab Twists - 3x30 seconds (1-2 minute rest inbetween sets)

Balance Workout 2

- Seated Ab Contractions - 3x8 (1-2 minute rest inbetween sets)
- Superman progression of your choice - 3x10 each side (1-2 minute rest inbetween sets)
- Static Shopping Bag Hold - 4x10 with 2 sec pauses (1-2 minute rest inbetween sets)
- Sit to Stand - 4x10 (2-3 minute rest inbetween sets)
- Glute Kickbacks - 3x10 (1-2 minute rest inbetween sets)

Balance Workout 3)

- Wood chops - 3x10 each side (1-2 minute rest inbetween sets)
- Ab Twists - 3x30 seconds (1-2 minute rest inbetween sets)
- Single Knee Raise and Tap - 3x10 each leg (1-2 minute rest inbetween sets)
- Squats - 3x10 (2-3 minute rest inbetween sets)
- Dead Bug progression of your choice - 3x10 each side (1-2 minute rest inbetween sets)

GENERAL STRENGTH, BALANCE AND MOBILITY WORKOUTS

The following workouts are great for improving your overall strength, balance and mobility as they are full body sessions that target many different muscle groups. Once you feel confident with your provided exercise plan you could eventually swap it out for these workouts, scheduling them at least 2-3 times each week to continue reaping the rewards of strength training!

All of the exercises in the workouts have been previously included in this book, if you're unsure on one of the exercises mentioned, please refer to the glossary at the back of this book to find the page number of each movement so that you can read step by step instructions, see the illustration or watch the video demonstration of the exercise.

These workouts start with the most accessible first.

Workout 1) (lying down)
- 10 and 2 Toes - 3x10 (1-2 minute rest inbetween sets)
- Chest Press - 3x10 (1-2 minute rest inbetween sets)
- Lying Leg Raise - 3x10 (1-2 minute rest inbetween sets)
- Clam Shells - 3x10 each side (1-2 minute rest inbetween sets)
- Arm Slides - 3x10 (1-2 minute rest inbetween sets)

Workout 2) (lying down)
- 10 and 2 toes - 3x10 (1-2 minute rest inbetween sets)

- Lying Lateral Leg Raise - 3x10 (1-2 minute rest inbetween sets)
- Clam Shells - 3x10 each side (1-2 minute rest inbetween sets)
- Single Leg Slides - 3x10 each side (1-2 minute rest inbetween sets)
- Single Arm Slides - 3x10 each side (1-2 minute rest inbetween sets)

Workout 3) (seated)

- Seated Heel Toes - 3x10 (1-2 minute rest inbetween sets)
- Seated Calf Raises - 3x10 (1-2 minute rest inbetween sets)
- Seated Leg Extensions - 3x10 (1-2 minute rest inbetween sets)
- Seated Military Press - 3x10 (1-2 minute rest inbetween sets)
- Seated Tricep Kickbacks - 3x10 (1-2 minute rest inbetween sets)

Workout 4) (seated)

- Seated Ab Contraction - 3x10 (1-2 minute rest inbetween sets)
- Seated Ab Twist - 3x10 each side (1-2 minute rest inbetween sets)
- Seated Calf Raises - 3x10 (1-2 minute rest inbetween sets)
- Seated Leg Curl - 3x10 (1-2 minute rest inbetween sets)
- Seated Bicep Curl - 3x10 each arm (1-2 minute rest inbetween sets)

Workout 5) (seated)

- Seated Ab Twist - 3x10 each side (1-2 minute rest inbetween sets)
- Seated Scapula Squeeze - 3x8 (1-2 minute rest inbetween sets)
- Seated Military Press - 3x10 (1-2 minute rest inbetween sets)
- Seated Calf Raise - 3x10 (1-2 minute rest inbetween sets)
- Seated Leg Extension - 3x0 (1-2 minute rest inbetween sets)

Workout 6 (seated)

- Seated Wood Chop - 3x10 each side (1-2 minute rest inbetween sets)

- Seated Ab Contraction - 3x10 each side (1-2 minute rest inbetween sets)
- Seated Leg Extension - 3x10 each leg (1-2 minute rest inbetween sets)
- Seated Leg Curl - 3x10 each leg (1-2 minute rest inbetween sets)
- Seated Arm Curl and Press - 3x10 (1-2 minute rest inbetween sets)

Workout 7 (seated)

- Seated March - 3x30 seconds (1-2 minute rest inbetween sets)
- Seated Leg Extensions - 3x10 each side (1-2 minute rest inbetween sets)
- Seated Horizontal Row - 3x10 (1-2 minute rest inbetween sets)
- Seated Svend Press - 3x10 (1-2 minute rest inbetween sets)
- Seated Heel-Toe Raises - 3x10 (1-2 minute rest inbetween sets)

Workout 8) (seated)

- Seated Heel-Toe Raises - 3x10 (1-2 minute rest inbetween sets)
- Seated Heel-Toes - 3x6 walkouts each side (1-2 minute rest inbetween sets)
- Seated Leg Extension - 3x10 (1-2 minute rest inbetween sets)
- Seated Leg Curl - 3x10 (1-2 minute rest inbetween sets)
- Seated Horizontal Row - 3x10 (1-2 minute rest inbetween sets)
- Seated Military Press - 3x10 (1-2 minute rest inbetween sets)

Workout 9)

- Seated March - 3x10 each leg (1-2 minute rest inbetween sets)
- Seated Ab Twist - 3x10 each side (1-2 minute rest inbetween sets)
- Glute Kick-Backs - 3x10 each side (2-3 minute rest inbetween sets)
- Supported Calf Raise (standing if possible) - 3x10 (1-2 minute rest inbetween sets)
- 1 Leg Balance - 3x8 each leg (1-2 minute rest inbetween sets)

Workout 10)

- Wood Chop - 3x10 each side (1-2 minute rest inbetween sets)
- Supported Single Leg Lifts - 3x10 each leg (1-2 minute rest inbetween sets)
- Standing Knee Lift and Tap - 3x10 each leg (1-2 minute rest inbetween sets)
- Sit to Stand - 3x10 (1-2 minute rest inbetween sets)
- Svend Press - 3x10 (1-2 minute rest inbetween sets)

Workout 11)

- Wood Chops - 3x10 each side (1-2 minute rest inbetween sets)
- Sit to Stands - 4x10 (2-3 minute rest inbetween sets)
- Seated Leg Extension - 3x10 (1-2 minute rest inbetween sets)
- Bent Over Row - 3x10 (1-2 minute rest inbetween sets)
- Military Press - 3x10 (1-2 minute rest inbetween sets)

Workout 12)

- Standing Knee Lift and Tap - 3x10 each side (1-2 minute rest inbetween sets)
- Shopping Bag Hold - 3x10 each side (1-2 minute rest inbetween sets)
- Ab Twists - 3x30 seconds (1-2 minute rest inbetween sets)
- Arm Curl and Overhead Press - 3x10 (1-2 minute rest inbetween sets)
- Bent Over Row - 3x10 (1-2 minute rest inbetween sets)

Workout 13)

- Standing Knee Lift and Tap - 3x10 each side (1-2 minute rest inbetween sets)
- Glute Kick-Backs - 3x10 each side (1-2 minute rest inbetween sets)
- Glute Bridge - 4x10 (2-3 minute rest inbetween sets)

- Push Up progression of your choice - 3x10 (1-2 minute rest inbetween sets)
- Lying Leg Raise - 3x10 (1-2 minute rest inbetween sets)

Workout 14)

- Ab Twists - 3x10 each side (1-2 minute rest inbetween sets)
- 1 Leg Balance - 3x10 each side (1-2 minute rest inbetween sets)
- Good Mornings - 3x10 (2-3 minute rest inbetween sets)
- Glute Kickbacks - 3x10 (1-2 minute rest inbetween sets)
- Chest Press - 3x10 (1-2 minute rest inbetween sets)

Workout 15)

- Superman progression of your choice - 3x10 each side (1-2 minute rest inbetween sets)
- Romanian Deadlifts - 3x10 (2-3 minute rest inbetween sets)
- Seated Leg Curl - 3x10 (1-2 minute rest inbetween sets)
- Military Press - 3x10 (1-2 minute rest inbetween sets)
- Seated Ab Contraction - 3x10 (1-2 minute rest inbetween sets)

Workout 16)

- Superman progression of your choice - 3x10 each side (1-2 minute rest inbetween sets)
- Floor Glute Kickbacks/Donkey Kicks - 3x10 each side (1-2 minute rest inbetween sets)
- Glute Bridge - 4x10 (2-3 minute rest inbetween sets)
- Military Press - 3x10 (1-2 minute rest inbetween sets)
- Bent Over Rows - 3x10 (1-2 minute rest inbetween sets)

Workout 17)

- Deadbug progression of your choice - 3x10 each side (1-2 minute rest inbetween sets)
- Lumbar Extensions - 3x10 (1-2 minute rest inbetween sets)
- Glute Bridge - 4x10 (2-3 minute rest inbetween sets)

- Chest Press - 3x10 (1-2 minute rest inbetween sets)
- Tricep Kickbacks - 3x10 (1-2 minute rest inbetween sets)

Workout 18)

- 1 Leg Balance - 8-10 each leg x3 (1-2 minute rest inbetween sets)
- Sit to Stands - 4x10 (2-3 minute rest inbetween sets)
- Chest Press - 3x10 (1-2 minute rest inbetween sets)
- Supported Calf Raises - 3x10 (1-2 minute rest inbetween sets)
- Push Ups - 3x10 (1-2 minute rest inbetween sets)

Workout 19)

- 4 Point Shoulder Taps - 3x10 each side (1-2 minute rest inbetween sets)
- Squats or Sit to Stands - 4x10 (2-3 minute rest inbetween sets)
- Bent Over Rows - 3x10 (1-2 minute rest inbetween sets)
- Chest Press - 3x10 (1-2 minute rest inbetween sets)
- Cat/Cow Stretch - 3x10 (1-2 minute rest inbetween sets)

Workout 20)

- Superman progression of your choice - 3x10 each side (1-2 minute rest inbetween sets)
- Shopping Bag Hold - 3x10 each side (1-2 minute rest inbetween sets)
- Romanian Deadlift - 4x10 (2-3 minute rest inbetween sets)
- Lying Leg Raise - 3x10 each leg (1-2 minute rest inbetween sets)
- Lumbar Extensions - 3x8-10 (1-2 minute rest inbetween sets)

Workout 21)

- Standing Knee Lift and Tap - 3x30 seconds alternating legs (1-2 minute rest inbetween sets)
- Squats - 4x10 (2-3 minute rest inbetween sets)
- Seated Leg Extension - 3x10 each leg (1-2 minute rest inbetween sets)

- Chest Press - 3x10 (1-2 minute rest inbetween sets)
- Tricep Kickbacks - 3x10 (1-2 minute rest inbetween sets)

Workout 22)

- Standing Knee Lift and Tap - 3x30 seconds alternating legs (1-2 minute rest inbetween sets)
- Romanian Deadlifts - 4x10 (2-3 minute rest inbetween sets)
- Glute Kick-backs - 3x10 each side (1-2 minute rest inbetween sets)
- Chest Press - 3x10 (1-2 minute rest inbetween sets)
- Tricep Kickbacks 3x10 (1-2 minute rest inbetween sets)

Workout 23)

- Superman progression of your choice - 3x10 each side (1-2 minute rest inbetween sets)
- Ab twists - 3x10 (1-2 minute rest inbetween sets)
- Squats - 4x10 (2-3 minute rest inbetween sets)
- Clam Shells - 3x10 each side (1-2 minute rest inbetween sets)
- Cat/Cow stretch - 3x10 (1-2 minute rest inbetween sets)

Workout 24)

- Dead Bug progression of your choice - 3x10 each side (1-2 minute rest inbetween sets)
- Good Mornings - 3x10 (2-3 minute rest inbetween sets)
- Lunges - 3x10 each side (2-3 minute rest inbetween sets)
- Chest Press - 3x10 (1-2 minute rest inbetween sets)
- Ab Twists - 3x10 each side (1-2 minute rest inbetween sets)

Workout 25)

- Sit to Stands - 3x10 (2-3 minute rest inbetween sets)
- Lunges - 3x10 (2-3 minute rest inbetween sets)
- 1 Leg Balance - 3x10 each side (1-2 minute rest inbetween sets)
- Lying Leg Raises - 3x10 (1-2 minute rest inbetween sets)

- Hamstring Stretch - 3x10 each side (1-2 minute rest inbetween sets)

Workout 26)

- Dead Bug progression of your choice - 3x10 each side (1-2 minute rest inbetween sets)
- Squats - 4x10 (2-3 minute rest inbetween sets)
- Supported Calf Raises - 3x10 (1-2 minute rest inbetween sets)
- Seated Ab Contraction 2x10 (1-2 minute rest inbetween sets)
- Lying Leg Raises - 3x10 (1-2 minute rest inbetween sets)

Workout 27)

- Wood Chop - 3x10 each side (1-2 minute rest inbetween sets)
- Sit to Stand - 4x10 (2-3 minute rest inbetween sets)
- Good Mornings - 3x10 (1-2 minute rest inbetween sets)
- Standing Knee Lift and Tap - 3x10 each side (1-2 minute rest inbetween sets)
- Ab Twists - 3x10 each side (1-2 minute rest inbetween sets)

Workout 28)

- Sit to Stand - 3x10 (1-2 minute rest inbetween sets)
- Lunges - 3x10 each leg (2-3 minute rest inbetween sets)
- Supported Calf Raise - 3x10 (1-2 minute rest inbetween sets)
- Lumbar Extensions - 3x10 (1-2 minute rest inbetween sets)
- Lateral Lying Leg Raises - 3x10 (1-2 minute rest inbetween sets)

Workout 29)

- Shopping Bag Carry - 6 lengths of the room (1-2 minute rest inbetween sets)
- Romanian Deadlifts - 3x10 (2-3 minute rest inbetween sets)
- Arm Curl and Overhead Press - 3x10 (1-2 minute rest inbetween sets)
- Svend Press - 3x10 (1-2 minute rest inbetween sets)

- Lumbar Extensions - 3x10 (1-2 minute rest inbetween sets)

Workout 30)

- Sit to Stand - 3x10 (1-2 minute rest inbetween sets)
- Lunges - 4x10 each leg (1-2 minute rest inbetween sets)
- Standing Knee Lift and Tap - 3x10 each leg (1-2 minute rest inbetween sets)
- Lying Lateral Leg Lifts - 3x10 each leg (1-2 minute rest inbetween sets)
- Lumbar Extensions - 3x10 (1-2 minute rest inbetween sets)

Summary

Now that you have a wealth of different exercises and workouts to try, as well as the knowledge on how to combine these exercises to make your own tailored workouts, you have all you need to become a stronger you!

Keep in mind that you can tailor each movement to your current ability and movements that may seem overwhelming and complicated now, could become easy with a few months of hard work and practice!

CONCLUSION

You can rise up from anything. You can completely recreate yourself. Nothing is permanent. You're not stuck. You have choices. You can think new thoughts. You can learn something new. You can create new habits. All that matters is that you decide today and never look back.

Idil Ahmed

No matter your age or fitness level, it's never too late to make a real difference in your life. Becoming more active is not just about adding years to your life but also about adding life to your years. I mean, who wants to live to a hundred if the last forty years are spent inactive or in pain?

Now that you'll be strength training regularly, you should soon feel stronger and more energetic. You'll be able to stay independent and continue enjoying the good things in life and will even look better on the outside, there's nothing like some blood flow to make the skin glow! Strength training can help protect your heart, boost your energy, and manage symptoms of sickness and pain, giving you a greater sense of well-being and helping you to enjoy your daily life that bit more.

Your new exercise routine will also be great for your mind, memory, and mood. No matter your age or physical condition, the tips and workouts shared in this book provide easy ways to become more active and improve your health and mindset and I just can't wait for you to reap the results of your hard work.

So often, we take our bodies for granted, but if we take a moment to be thankful for all our body does – not only walking and moving around but even breathing and healing – the gratitude would be never-ending. In truth, your body is a unique healing machine, intricately designed and wonderfully made! And your task now is to maintain it.

Though one classification of age is chronological, other factors such as lifestyle and environment also have significant effects. This means that the number of years you've lived does not need to be equal to your fitness, mobility, or health. Of course, it will have an effect, but hundreds of thousands of seniors worldwide live long, healthy, fit lives, and you're now on your way to being one of them!

If you stay consistent with your strength training routine and remember to nourish your body with balanced foods, you could now have more time with your family, go on unforgettable holidays, watch your grandkids grow up, and be independent for as long as you live without being limited by fragility and pain. Life's too short for anything other than pain free happiness.

My deepest hope is that you use the strength training plan and exercises in this book to form a new lifestyle. We've discussed the amazing benefits of exercise for your body, brain, and soul and you now have all the tools you need to get and stay strong. I hope strength training is as life changing for you as it has been for me.

Most importantly, please don't forget to enjoy your journey, take it one day at a time and remember to praise your body for the incredible machine that it is! I wish you so much strength, energy and confidence and I KNOW you can have it all. You've got this, happy training!

GLOSSARY

A Quick Note!

If you enjoyed this book I'd really appreciate it if you'd leave a review on Amazon!

Reviews really help independent writers like myself get in front of the right audience and help more people!

If you have any constructive feedback, or anything you'd really like to see in a future book, please let me know at sophie@ strongandstretchy.co.uk.

Thank you so much in advance!

REFERENCES

[i] https://www.registerednursing.org/articles/healthcare-costs-by-age/

Bucceri Androus, RN, BSN, A. (2021). Here's how much your healthcare costs will rise as you age. *You're Going to Need a Lot of Money for Your Healthcare Costs When You're Older.*

[ii] https://www.sciencedaily.com/releases/2016/04/160420090406.htm

Strength training helps older adults live longer. (2016). ScienceDaily.

[iii] https://www.statista.com/statistics/1222815/loneliness-among-adults-by-country/#:~:text=Feeling%20of%20loneliness%20among%20adults%202021%2C%20by%20country&text=According%20to%20a%20global%-20survey,often%2C%20always%2C%20or%20sometimes.

Statista. (2021, November 4). *Feeling of loneliness among adults 2021, by country.* https://www.statista.com/statistics/1222815/loneliness-among-adults-by-country/#:%7E:text=Feeling%20of%20loneliness%20among%20adults%202021%2C%20by%20country&text=According%20to%20a%20global%20survey,often%2C%20always%2C%20or%20sometimes.

[iv] https://knowablemagazine.org/article/mind/2022/exercise-boosts-brain-mental-health

Holmes. (2022). *Exercise boosts the brain — And mental health.* Knowable Magazine.

[v]   https://www.sydney.edu.au/news-opinion/news/2020/02/11/strength-training-can-help-protect-the-brain-from-degeneration.html#:~:text=Researchers%20have%20found%20that%20six,up%20to%20one%20year%20later.&text=The%20hippocampus%20is%20a%20complex,role%20in%20learning%20and%20memory

Strength training can help protect the brain from degeneration. (2020). *The University of Sydney.*

[vi] https://www.menshealth.com/uk/building-muscle/a31285357/muscle-old-age/

Lane, E. (2021, January 18). *Over 60? You Can Still Build New Muscle Well Into Your 70s, Says Science.* Men's Health. https://www.menshealth.com/uk/building-muscle/a31285357/muscle-old-age/

[vii] https://pubmed.ncbi.nlm.nih.gov/22760906/

Is exercise an alternative treatment for chronic insomnia? (2012). *National Library of Medicine.*

[viii] https://www.sciencedaily.com/releases/2020/06/200615115725.htm

Multi-ethnic study suggests vitamin K may offer protective health benefits in older age: Older adults with low vitamin K had higher death risk over 13 years compared to those with adequate vitamin K levels. (2020). ScienceDaily. https://www.sciencedaily.com/releases/2020/06/200615115725.htm

[ix] https://www.everydayhealth.com/fitness/add-strength-training-to-your-workout.aspx#:~:text=Strength%20Training%20Helps%20You%20Develop%20Better%20Body%20Mechanics&text=%E2%80%9CBalance%20

is%20dependent%20on%20the,%2C%20the%20better%20 your%20balance.%E2%80%9D

Iliades, C., MD, & Cutler, D. M. O., PhD. (2021, October 5). *The Benefits of Strength and Weight Training.* EverydayHealth. Com. https://www.everydayhealth.com/fitness/add-strength-training-to-your-workout.aspx#:%7E:text=Strength%20 Training%20Helps%20You%20Develop%20Better%20 Body%20Mechanics&text=%E2%80%9CBalance%20 is%20dependent%20on%20the,%2C%20the%20better%20 your%20balance.%E2%80%9D

Additional Resources:

- https://thriva.co/hub/wellness/nose-breathing-benefits

  T. (2022). *6 reasons why nose breathing is important.* Thriva - Track and Improve Your Health. https://thriva.co/hub/wellness/ nose-breathing-benefits
- https://loaids.com/senior-fitness-quotes/

  L. (2021, June 24). *50 Inspiring Senior Fitness Quotes To Keep You Moving.* Loaids.
- https://www.nhs.uk/common-health-questions/womens-health/ what-are-pelvic-floor-exercises/

  NHS website. (2021, November 30). *What are pelvic floor exercises?* NHS.Uk.
- https://www.health.harvard.edu/staying-healthy/strength-training-builds-more-than-muscles

  Strength Training Builds More than Muscles. (2021). Harvard.Edu.
- https://www.arthritis-health.com/blog/strength-training-can-crush-arthritis-pain?fbclid=IwAR0eMPXvTYdwGRNs5Hy8cB E2RfX5ZbFnaoYd5kKuUtvoP0TWg3SFBaNNq1Q
- DeVries, C. (2015). *Strength Training Can Crush Arthritis Pain.* Arthritis-Health. https://www.arthritis-health.com/blog/ strength-training-can-crush-arthritis-pain?fbclid=IwAR0eMPXv

TYdwGRNs5Hy8cBE2RfX5ZbFnaoYd5kKuUtvoP0TWg3SFB
aNNq1Q

- Treanor, M. (2022). *Picture Quotes*. PictureQuotes.Com. http://
  www.picturequotes.com/exercise-not-only-tones-the-muscles-
  but-also-refines-the-brain-and-revives-the-soul-quote-213382

www.ingramcontent.com/pod-product-compliance
Lightning Source LLC
Chambersburg PA
CBHW050723030426
42336CB00012B/1400